# A TEN MINUTE CURE FOR THE COMMON COLD

## A Natural Approach

*JAMES F. DOROBIALA, D.C.*

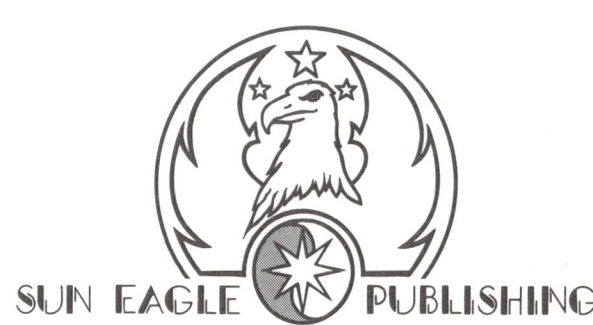

Granada Hills, California

© 1988 - James F. Dorobiala, D.C.
First Edition published in 1988 by
Sun Eagle Publishing
P.O. Box 33545
Granada Hills, CA 91344-8545

ALL RIGHTS RESERVED
No part of this book may be reproduced, translated, or transmitted in any form by any means electronic or mechanical including photocopy without written permission from the publisher. Reviewers may quote brief passages.

Library of Congress Cataloging-in-Publication Data

Dorobiala, James F., 1941-
   a ten minute cure for the common cold.

   Bibliography: pp. 168
   Includes index.
     1. Cold (Disease)—Treatment.
     2. Naturopathy.
   I. Title.
   RF361.D67 1987     616.2 ' 0506     87-18114
     ISBN 0-944346-01-4 (hardcover)
     ISBN 0-944346-02-2 (softcover)
     ISBN 0-944346-03-0 (tape) VHS
     ISBN 0-944346-05-7 (tape) BETA

Printed in the United States of America

## CATCHING COLD?

At last there is something effective you can do to uncatch it. The <u>Ten Minute Cure For The Common Cold</u> is the New Age answer to what has been considered virtually untreatable. Put an end to the annual coughing, hacking, sneezing, and sniveling.

Hundreds of varieties of rhinoviruses are on the prowl in fall and winter, corona viruses in late winter, and adenoviruses in early spring. These are the major culprits which cause common cold miseries. Summer colds are often attributed to parainfluenza viruses or enteroviruses which complete the year round cycle of suffering.

The typical individual sneezes and coughs his way through six colds a year. On the average six days of work or school are lost and many other days are written off as hardly worth living. Unnecessary illness is monetarily expensive and physically and psychologically debilitating. Potions and over the counter nostrums which may not result in any real benefit only add to the cost and may cause harmful side effects.

A <u>Ten Minute Cure For The Common Cold</u> is currently the only definitive work available on cure and management of the common cold. Master the work presented in this book and demonstrated on the video tape! By doing so, you have chosen to maintain good health and not to participate in the needless prolonged common cold syndrome.

Publisher's Note: The information presented here is the result of years of research. Other research may indicate different results or produce differing opinions. The author does not intend this book to be used to treat physical conditions that should be handled by a competent, trained professional.

Adequate and diligent preparation has gone into the explanation of how to safely practice all techniques presented in this work. Neither the author nor the publisher accepts any responsibility for any problems real or imagined which may arise from misapplication of the techniques herein presented.

For legal reasons as well as professional courtesy we must recommend that you follow your doctor's advice in all health matters relating to yourself or those you may wish to assist.

**WARNING:** Movement of bones is not necessary in any of the procedures outlined in this book. To do so without proper training can be dangerous. Do not attempt to move the bones in the spinal column unless you are licensed to do so. All licensed health care practitioners may incorporate these methods as appropriate to their particular specialties within the legal constraints of their scope of practice.

# FOREWORD

In a TEN MINUTE CURE FOR THE COMMON COLD, Dr. James Dorobiala offers a procedure hitherto unavailable to patients at large.

How many physicians have presented you with a way to prevent a cold or nip it at the first onset of symptoms? Without harmful drugs?

Remember this: there is no reason to get colds. People who take care of themselves naturally choosing a positive mental outlook, proper diet and exercise are virtually cold-free (or free of fractionally any disease for that matter). And if they should on rare occasions become upset or rundown or unduly exposed to the elements, using Dr. Dorobiala's techniques, they can get back on the track in a nick of time. No harmful chemicals, no doctor's bills, no absenteeism. In addition, anyone who successfully learns to look after himself get the added benefit of feeling that he is in control, that he can manage his health and keep on course toward his chosen goals. He stays on top of it; he's a winner!

Health, Oriental Medicine teaches us, is a matter of energetic balance. That is not just a theory. Access to the "energetic switches" that monitor that energy balance are right there on your body, in specific locations called "points". Press lightly, and a subtle yet powerful reflex through certain brain centers to the immune system or organs in need is triggered immediately. Since prolonged energetic imbalance leads to functional trouble and later on to tissue damage, treating yourself energetically and keeping yourself fit at those fine levels makes a lot more sense that waiting for chemical suppressants or the surgeon's knife. Have you ever tried doing a good day's work on anti-histamines or codeine?

Then, what about homeopathics? Isn't that "taking

pills"? No. Homeopathics are not chemical pills in the traditional sense. They are "frequential" pills, i.e. they retain and transmit only the frequential properties of certain vegetable, mineral or animal substances without their chemicals properties — or a trace amount occasionally depending on the potency. Their ingestion effects an immediate energetic or frequential change necessary to reverse the disease frequencies - causing disturbance in the body. That is why homeopathic tablets are taken under the tongue onto the delicate and highly absorptive sub-glossal mucosa from where in three seconds their medicinal property will make its way through the blood stream to the cells. Low potencies, as recommended in Dr. Dorobiala's book, cause no aggravations of symptoms and act quickly. Modern European research in homeopathy clearly makes it the medicine of the future in general practice; so, do not be deflected in your quest for better health, by the retrograde opinions of certain dinosaurian minds who relegate homeopathy to the rank of a placebo. Double blind studies conducted jointly by the Glasgow Homeopathic Hospital, the Department of Bacteriology and Immunology and the Department of Statistics of the University of Glasgow and published in the prestigious British medical journal, The Lancet (October, 1986) clearly repudiate the established allopathic belief that homeopathy is not medicinal.

Finally, in an age dazzled by wild technological prodigies, few realize that when it comes to measuring the human energy field, even the slightest voltage given off by an electrical instrument may disrupt the very field one needs to assess. Lately, certain German instrumentation has become quite sophisticated, but still lacking and at any rate out of range for the average patient. Therefore; the human bodymind, the most sophisticated agency on earth, is used both as an instrument and as a witness to access the information needed. Pressing a positive diagnostic point makes a strong muscle reflexively go weak. Introducing within the field a correcting frequency — in the form of the appropriate homeopathic remedy or the right meridian point — makes the muscle regain its strength. A simple law of re-adjusting frequencies; not magic, not witchcraft. And not harmful.

Applied correctly and within the paradigms outlined by Dr. Dorobiala, the method will be of great help to many. At a time of unsafe allopathic drugs, inflated healthcare costs, James Dorobiala's research and contribution is inspiring and will go a long way toward helping those in need of a ten-minute cure for their aggravating and how-unnecessary common cold.

Marc LeBel, OMD
Past Dean, California Acupuncture College
Los Angeles, California

# ABOUT THE AUTHOR

Dr. Dorobiala grew up on the cold damp shores of Lake Ontario in Upstate New York. He was at an early age no stranger to colds, flues, and allergies. At age 15, after almost dying of anaphalactic shock due to an ill-advised allergy injection, he vowed to find a way to end this triad of misery in a natural way. This vow was, however, some years in fulfillment. First came a Bachelor of Arts Degree in Modern Languages; three years in the U.S. Army during the Vietnam conflict; Bachelor of Foreign Trade degree and a Masters Degree in International Management.

He spent five years in the Far East as an Operations Officer with one of New York's leading financial institutions. Living in the Far East afforded the opportunity of studying local Asian folk healing techniques. After returning from Asia he enrolled in the Los Angeles College of Chiropractic where he graduated in 1978. While in school he was awarded the James Parker Scholarship, and the 1978 John A. Fisher Memorial Scholarship for the Most Outstanding Chiropractic College Senior in the United States.

He holds a teaching credential for California Community Colleges in Health Sciences and is an extension faculty member for his alma mater. He is currently Director of Education and Research with the American Academy of Holistic Chiropractic and is listed in the First Edition of International Who's Who in Medicine.

Dr. Dorobiala is Director of North Valley Chiropractic Clinic in Granada Hills, California which he established in 1979. He devotes much of his time to Chiropractic and para-related research on the natural cure of illnesses. In addition to advanced Chiropractic he has studied

Homeopathy, Zone Therapy, Reflexology, Scientific Massage, Accupressure, Auricular Medicine, and Crystal healing techniques. He is the developer of Advanced Regenerative Chiropractic Technique. Dr. Dorobiala is a student and practitioner of the internal martial art systems-Tai Chi Chuan, Hsing-I, and Pa Kua Chang—all of which deal with the accumulation and application of Chi/Ki energy for health and physical fitness as well as self defense.

## ACKNOWLEDGEMENTS

To my wife Michelle who encouraged me to write this book; to my children Christina, Andrea, Aarik and Michael who supplied me regularly with fresh colds upon which to work. Drs. Ted Ronyon, D.C., Victor Frank, D.C., the late Hal Havlik, D.C., Robert Deutsch, D.C., and Donald Dossey, Ph.D., all of whom played a significant part in my educational background and motivated me to research and publish my findings. To my many loyal patients who gave me the numerical exposure to cold virus cases to prove that the system works. To Mssrs. Minh Luong and Larry S. Day whose illustrations appear through-out this volume as noted. To Mssrs. Quang and Phan Luong for photography and technical assistance. To Kerry A. Martinez for proof reading and editing. To Eleanor and Don Biggs, Eric and Carrie Fable for their constructive review commentary. Also Larry S. Day for assistance with graphics and cover design.

## DEDICATION

"To the eradication of the watering eye, runny nose, explosive sneeze, hacking cough and scratchy throat."

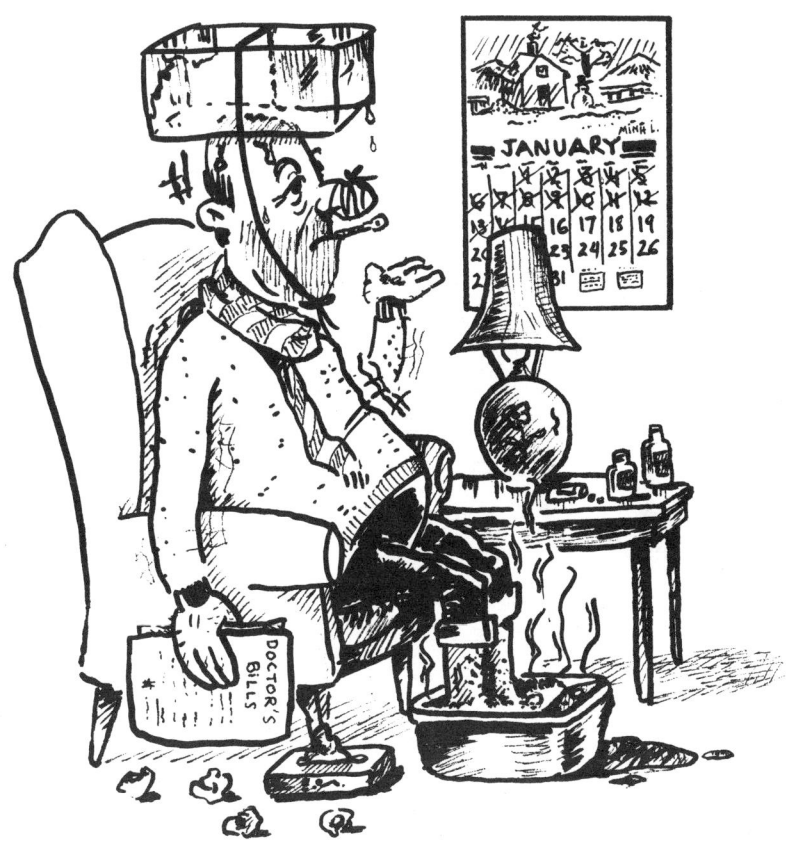

## TABLE OF CONTENTS

| | | |
|---|---|---|
| I | INTRODUCTION | 1 |
| II | DEFINITIONS | 5 |
| III | VIRUSES AND THE IMMUNE SYSTEM | 11 |
| IV | A WORKING THEORY | 13 |
| V | PREREQUISITES FOR A POSITIVE OUTCOME | 23 |
| VI | APPLICATION OF THE TECHNIQUE | 27 |
| VII | TESTING PROCEDURES FOR THE HANDICAPPED, BEDRIDDEN, YOUNG CHILDREN AND INFANTS | 63 |
| VIII | CHEST COLDS & SORE THROATS | 69 |
| IX | REFLEXOLOGY AND ZONE THERAPY | 81 |
| X | NUTRITIONAL SUGGESTIONS | 95 |
| XI | TESTING VITAMINS, MINERALS, AND OTHER CHEMICAL SUBSTANCES | 99 |
| XII | HELPFUL HOMEOPATHIC REMEDIES | 103 |

| XIII | HOW TO FIND AND TEST FOR APPROPRIATE REMEDY(S), POTENCY, AND DOSAGE INTERVAL | 113 |
| --- | --- | --- |
| XIV | CLEANSING THE NASAL PASSAGES AND SINUSES | 119 |
| XV | EPILOGUE | 125 |
| XVI | SELF HELP PRODUCT LIST | 129 |
| XVII | RECOMMENDED READING | 133 |
| | APPENDIX I — DIAGRAMS & PHOTOGRAPHS | 137 |
| | APPENDIX II — PROCEDURAL FLOW CHART | 143 |
| | INDEX | 147 |

# CHAPTER I: INTRODUCTION

To paraphrase an old English medical proverb, it was said that, "a cold usually lasts 14 days if treated and a fortnight if not." Fortunately, due to recent Chiropractic research, this need not be the case. The time missed from work, school and social engagements is well near incalculable on a worldwide basis due to the variety of nefarious cold viruses. Even after a cold has run its course, it often leaves one weakened and prone to residuals such as sinusitus, bronchitis, and pneumonia, just to name a few well known miseries.

Some health enthusiasts have convinced themselves that a cold is our friend and is only nature's way of house cleaning our badly mistreated physical bodies. While there is some truth to this premise, my experience as a Chiropractic physician and Homeopathic practitioner leads me to view the cold as nothing more than a pathology. Rather than waiting for the virus to digest all the accumulated toxins lodged in a body, thereby ultimately starving itself to death which is the probable reason why colds tend to be self limiting, we should look to a method where ultra rapid acceleration of this natural process can be accomplished. This can be done through systematic technique. The "Ten Minute Cure" opens blocked energy channels, restores proper body polarity and assists the liver in rapid detoxification. With nothing left to eat the virus dies with no time to create allergic conditions in the body. I have in the course of practice effected this result countless times. You the reader, by digesting and applying the material which you are about to read will reproduce the very same results, thus freeing yourself, your patients and loved ones from the miseries of the common cold.

This book was written principally for anyone and everyone interested in getting rid of colds. I have endeavored to use fairly nontechnical language to that end. What I propose to present in the following pages is a simple, concise, effective method of dealing with the common cold. Almost anyone with average intelligence, a measure of patience, and just a mustard seed of faith and belief can master this system. The results will be well worth the effort expended. This is a "hands on" book geared toward results—not a dialectic position to be attacked, defended or argued. For the sake of grammatical efficiency all reference and usage of the pronoun "his" is to be construed to mean "his/her" as appropriate.

All techniques presented have evolved through clinical experience over a seven year period. Positive results are consistently reproducible by systematic step-by-step application of these simple procedures. Although the technique was developed through Chiropractic research, it stands on its own merit as a unique form of accupressure and can be readily incorporated into any rational healing art form.

# DEFINITIONS

# CHAPTER II: DEFINITIONS

A. Virus: comes from Latin and signifies:

    1. Slime, poison, stench, that which corrupts ; an evil influence.
    2. Any of a group of ultra or submicroscopic infective agents that cause disease.

B. Cure: Comes from middle English and old French "cure"—Latin "Cura."

    1. A healing, the act of healing, restoration to health.
    2. A remedy, that which makes one well.
    3. A system or method of treatment.

C. Patient: Comes from the Latin "pati" to suffer.

    1. Someone who has encountered "A" and has need of "B."
    2. A person receiving care or treatment.

## CHAPTER II: DEFINITIONS

D. Accu-digipressure: A method of gentle vibrational stimulation of the nervous system accomplished with the thumbs or fingers by rythmic circular pressure on specific bladder meridian points above and adjacent to the spinal vertebra. Kinetic movement of the individual segments is not a requirement for successful implementation.

E. Bladder Meridian: For our purposes this is an invisible energy channel which runs bilaterally parallel to the spinal column from the base of the skull to the sacrum.

F. Muscle Testing: A process whereby a specific muscle group is challenged for integrity (strength) so that it may be used as an indicator of normal or aberrant function in a physical body.

G. Joint Lock: A marginal range of motion of 5-20° created when opposing muscular forces of healer and patient reach the relative neutralization point during the muscle testing procedure.

H. Witness: Any physical, spoken, or written energy component which signifies a pathogenic entity or curative element.

I. Circuit A: Testing patient in open handed posture.

J. Circuit B: Testing patient in thumb/pinky configuration.

K. Testing in the "clear":

1. Testing an intact muscle (circuit A) against any reflex point or witness; weakness to be corrected by specific segmental stimulation as described in steps I - VI.

2. Patient is in open handed posture or in thumb/pinky configuration. Focuses circuit A or B as required.

3. Testing any specific muscle or muscle group without touching the body reflex points or employing a witness. Muscle weakness must be corrected before administering the Ten Minute Cure.

4. Testing vitamins, minerals, herbs, homeopathic remedies or drugs against the body's electro magnetic energy field without contacting specific reflex points.

L. Phase one correction:

1. Testing circuit A in the clear against the witness or specific reflex points has demonstrated deficiency by muscle weakness.

2. Stimulation of circuit A bladder meridian points in the presence of a witness by specific formulae (i.e. T2,5,8 - Liver).

3. Stimulation of circuit A bladder meridian points without the presence of the witness by specific formula (i.e. T1,5,9 - Spleen). Patient or healer touches spleen point while testing is accomplished-not while correction is made.

4. Employing digital stimulation to antibiotic, cold and sinus meridian points.

5. Patient is in open handed posture.

M. Phase two correction:

1. Stimulation of circuit A vertebral segment bladder meridian points with the presence of a witness while the patient holds specific reflex points.

2. Stimulation of circuit A bladder meridian points without the presence of the witness. In steps four and five the witness is withdrawn and the patient holds specific reflex points.

3. Performed in lieu of phase one correction if the patient is obviously symptomatic and testing in the clear demonstrates no muscle weakness for phase one challenge.

4. Patient is in open handed posture.

5. In step four and five the witness is withdrawn and the patient holds specific reflex points while vertebral levels that indicate strength are stimulated.

N. Phase three correction:

1. Stimulation of circuit B spinal segment bladder meridian points as in phase two correction except hand contacts reflex points with the thumb and pinky joined.

2. Performed after phase two correction and circuit A has been reintergrated.

3. In step four and five the witness is withdrawn and the patient holds specific reflex points while vertebral levels that perpetuate weakness are stimulated.

O. Segmental or Vertebral circuitry:

1. Sub-circuits which are governed by individual vertebra.

2. Circuits which function within the scope of circuit A or B depending upon which is being focused.

3. Circuits which reach out to the organ/glandular systems of the body via the spinal column.

4. Circuits which are accessed and corrected through phase one, two, and three testing and stimulation procedures.

5. Circuits which interface with bladder meridian points.

# CHAPTER III:
# VIRUSES AND THE IMMUNE SYSTEM

The Germ Theory simply stated says that disease is caused by microbacteria and viruses which gang up and pounce on you overpowering your resistance. Either you catch them or they catch you. A great battle goes on between you and the invaders. If you are the stronger, you get well and live; if not you get sick and die. This of course would be the extreme case. This theory is rapidly being replaced in many scientific circles with the Immune System Deficiency Syndrome model. This theory entertains the idea that germs and viruses are present around and in us almost all the time anyway, and that we fall ill due to the integrity of our immune systems. This means that if our immune system is weak, then germs and viruses get a foothold and get about their nasty business of making us miserable. There is much to be said for this line of reasoning.

What weakens our immune systems? Some people are born with immune system deficiencies. A breast-fed baby born of a healthy mother has a far better chance of developing a sound immune system than one who gets only a manufactured formula. Other reasons are fairly obvious: bad eating habits, inadequate rest, ecological pollution. Emotional stress of modern living makes us feel older than our years.

Some people seem to be more constitutionally prone to "take cold" than others. No one likes to dance the "Sneezer's Waltz." How many times have you been unfortunate enough to be the unwilling target of a misty sneeze when packed in a stuffy elevator, or watched the waiter or waitress fumble for a hanky to stem a runny nose as you were brought your prime rib dinner. It was just a matter of time before your nose resembled a leaky faucet. A handkerchief is contaminated by what it touches, and contaminates everything and everyone that touches it. Never borrow someones hanky if you want to stay healthy!

One day as I was doing some research on the Chiropractic cure of allergy, it dawned on me that the common cold could be effectively treated in much the same way with positive results, without heavy patent medications and undesirable side effects. Many medical doctors routinely prescribe antibiotics for the common cold knowing full well that viruses are essentially unaffected by them. The antibiotic may be effective only against a so called secondary opportunistic infection which may follow a viral invasion.

Problems arise when ingested antibiotics kill all the intestinal flora; friendly bacteria necessary to good health, as well as the bad. Many times a culture and sensitivity is not done by the physician and the routinely prescribed antibiotic is totally ineffective against the pathogen. This often paves the way for a systemic "yeastlike fungus infection" of the species Candida Albicans. The USA is suffering an epidemic of Candida overgrowth, as well as other related species, mainly due to indiscriminant administration of antibiotics.

Please don't misunderstand—antibiotics have their proper place in the healing profession and should be reserved for serious or life threatening occassions. Chicken and domestic fowl lovers are especially prone to Candida overgrowth because of the forced feeding with antibiotic laced grain generally practiced by commercial industry. This is another contributor to a weakened immune system. Fowl and swine are very susceptible to viruses themselves. Forced antibiotic feeding should be stopped. It is a violation of nature, and the negative effects on the human immune system are far reaching.

The effect of the perpetual presence of antibiotics in human and animal ecosystems is antibiotic resistent strains of bacteria that do not respond to the very means that created them; namely, antibiotic therapy!

# CHAPTER IV:
# A WORKING THEORY

The human brain is without a doubt the most sophisticated bio-computer available on the planet. Scientists say that we are only using 5-10% of its capacity. Looking at the current state of world affairs, one wonders what would happen if more were available to us given our retarded state of social evolution. Be that as it may, it is the subconscious function that apparently runs the physical body. You normally don't have to remember to breathe. If you did, life would be most difficult to say the least.

Under normal circumstances, given a good diet, decent heredity patterns, and a balanced mental/emotional outlook which appropriately responds to the routine stresses of living, a reasonable state of health is maintained. When any of these factors is out of balance, disease or ill health is the outcome. It is not my intent to present detailed explanations of the complicated immune system response to something the body considers a threat to its well-being. Even a pretty rose may be considered an enemy and cause an allergic reaction. This is an example of inappropriate antibody/immune system reaction to a generally harmless flower. It suffices to say that the cold virus, in its various forms, is an ancient organism and has been around at least as long as man on the planet. It has managed to survive rather well despite being dosed with a barrage of chemical substances and vile curses.

To stretch the imagination a bit, let's credit the cold virus with having a sort of primitive, yet highly sophisticated intelligence factor geared to it's survival. It is generally accepted that the cold virus enters a victim's body through the oral/nasal passages via vehicles such as sneezing, coughing, kissing, and hand to mouth contamination. Once in the body, the virus in its desire to survive and replicate, effects certain physiological changes.

How does a virus get into a cell? First, let's examine what a virus is. A virus consists of a small number of genes made up of DNA/RNA molecules. It wears a protective coat of protein which has spikes sticking out from its outer surface which allows it to interface with a host cell of its choice. It may masquerade as a hormone or other molecule that the cell ordinarily has need of and would normally take right in without question. Viruses are 10 to 100 times smaller than the average bacteria; much smaller than the wavelength of visible light. They can be detected only by a fairly recent invention, the electron microscope. X-ray crystallography reveals the cold virus to resemble a soccer ball with a lumpy protein surface of triangular facets.

Once inside the trusting body cell, no more Mr. Nice Guy! The virus dumps its genetic material into the ready cellular cytoplasm. The foreign genes hijack the cell's machinery to redirect its function into making carbon copies of themselves. It spreads like wildfire. Of course this finally alerts the immune system to produce T-cells and appropriate antibodies, but this does the cold sufferer little good in the short run. Antibodies in the blood may

## CHAPTER IV: A WORKING THEORY

not get to the cells where they are needed. Viruses have an amazing ability to mutate, which may explain why no lasting immunity to colds has been acquired by the general population. By the time an antibody has been formed to search out an invader, the virus may have donned another disguise and slipped through the immunological dragnet. Then too, there are a vast number of different strains of the virus which one has never before encountered.

This ingenious process begins shorting out certain switches in your personal bio-computer. Usually the liver is the first to be affected. The immune system is unable to respond appropriately due to a series of short circuits. It reacts in an allergic manner to the viral toxins which are biproducts of virus life cycle activity. The result is a symptomalogical response called "a cold."

Viruses will feed upon or digest toxins which have accumulated and blocked certain points in the accupuncture energy meridians. The natural path of the body's electomagnetic odic or pranic force becomes distorted causing a shift in polarity. This polarity shift makes it easy for the virus to proliferate.

A word about fever: Fever is the body's natural attempt to "burn out" toxins and open the energy channels. It also attempts to change the thermal parameters within which a virus can survive. Temperatures under 104°F for a day or two are helpful and should not be "lowered" with aspirin. Cool sponge or alcohol baths are far superior in this respect. Prolongued temperatures over 104°F can alter brain protein composition. Temperature this high are usually due to some other infectious organism and will warrant a different form of therapy. It is likely antibiotics would be required.

People often respond to this energy field distortion according to a constitutional type or inherent genetic weakness. This is to say, some are prone to head colds, others chest colds, for others it settles in the throat. The location really doesn't matter. The approach is ever the same and the results predictable. One must determine which switches have been inactivated by the viral legions and reactivate them. This restores the bio-computer to full capacity which corrects the aberrant immune response and brings balance once again to the system. To lower toxic residues in the body is to lower virus survival potential. Sounds easy doesn't it? It really is, but the procedure must be done in a specific manner in order to produce the desired effect.

To do this we must ask the bio-computer which circuits have been deactivated. This is accomplished by simple kinesiological or muscle testing procedures. The bio-computer is set up on a binary "yes" or "no" programming. The subconscious is generally aware of what is wrong with the body at all times, even if it is not able to fix it. By asking it via muscle response symbolism (weak or strong) the desired information can be obtained.

The next step is to determine if the affliction is a flu virus, allergic reaction to a different alien substance, or the cold virus itself. This is done through a working knowledge of simple test points and a witness or specimen representing the nature of the inquiry.

This can be done via a small piece of blotter paper soaked in a cold victim's saliva and a plastic bag, or by simply writing the name of the pathogen on a piece of paper. The latter method is least messy and is made possible through the <u>Universal Law of Harmonic Correspondences</u> which simply stated says:

> "the essence of a person, place or thing resonates in a vibratory manner throughout the material, emotional and mental spheres of existence."

## CHAPTER IV: A WORKING THEORY

Words are merely symbolic containers for ideas or thought forms. Thoughts are living things! Therefore, by writing the words "Your Cold Virus" on a piece of paper and introducing it into a person's electromagnetic field (or aura) which connects to the bio-computer, the reaction will be the same as if you presented a biological specimen of cold virus to the body. Research has demonstrated the body's ability to read and process symbolic information. I have tried both methods many times and find the processes to be consistent and interchangeable. However, if you have a mental resistance to the piece of paper routine, you may rely solely on the saliva blotter paper method. However, do write "Your Cold Virus" on the blotter paper before saturating. Keep the ink or pencil impression dry. You may also wish to include a cotton swab with nasal secretions to be tested together or separately. Viral concentration is extremely high in nasal secretions, much more so than in saliva.

You must identify precisely the condition you wish to treat. Then alert the body to accept the treatment. A working knowledge of the human spine, bladder meridian points and some specific test points is necessary. The normal spinal column is comprised of the neck or 7 cervical segments - the upper back or 12 dorsal/thoracic segments - the lower back or 5 lumbar segments, and at the very tip of the spine the sacrum and coccyx (Figure 2). These will be your landmarks with respect to identifying and reactivating faulty computer switches. Learn them well!

Passing out from the spinal column which connects to the brain/bio-computer are spinal nerves. They flow out to the various organs and endocrine functions which must be corrected and reenergized. Proper stimulation of the bladder meridian points adjacent to these spinal vertebra will render the cold virus and its physical effects harmless. We are essentially altering conditions in the body; creating an atmosphere in which a virus cannot function.

Lastly, familiarize yourself (Figures 3, 4, & 10 ) with the cold test point located on the fleshy palmer mount at the base of the thumb on both hands. Then the liver, thymus, spleen, throat, pituitary (master gland), sinus, lung, bronchi reflex points, and the natural antibiotic point (Figure 5). These are essentially all you will need to know to deal with the average cold attack.

A convenient way to locate specific spinal reference vertebrae is as follows:

1. Tip the patient's head gently back into extension. You will notice a depression or deep indentation at the base of the skull. If you put your thumb into it you will have located the second cervical vertebra.

2. Counting downward you will come to a large protruding vertebra at the base of the neck. This is usually the first dorsal vertebra, but on some patients may be the seventh cervical segment. Counting the spinous processes (bumps on the spine) individually from C2 will facilitate proper identification.

3. Place a straight edge across the lower tips of the shoulder blades (scapulae). It will cross the spine at the bottom of 7th dorsal vertebra (T7).

4. Place a straight edge across the crests of the Ilia (top of the hip bones). It will cross the spine at the level of the 4th lumbar vertebra (L4).

5. The bladder meridian points will be found on the skin

surface over the tips of the tranverse processes of the spinal vertebra.

Counting upward or downward from any of the reference points will permit you to identify any specific vertebra with relative ease.

# CHAPTER V: PREREQUISITES FOR A POSITIVE OUTCOME:

1. An open mind.

2. The intent to heal; an act of Universal Love.

3. Faith, confidence and belief in one's self.

4. Learning simple muscle testing procedures.

5. A working knowledge of the spinal column and bladder meridian points.

6. Specific reflex points:

   a. Liver     b. Thymus

   c. Spleen    d. Hand cold points

   e. Sinus     f. Lungs

## CHAPTER V: PREREQUISITES FOR A POSITIVE OUTCOME

    g. Bronchi   h. Antibiotic points

7. A piece of blotter paper, cotton swabs, pen or pencil, and a plastic bag.

8. Your thumbs and index finger or middle fingers.

9. A Homeopathic Test Kit.

10. Two homeopathic remedies; Aconite and Nux Vomica.

11. Two effervescent bicarbonate of soda tablets; without aspirin for children or those who have aspirin allergy. These items are optional but extremely helpful. Omit for patients with heart problems or sodium restricted diets.

    The cure is based upon reflex principles via stimulation of spinal nerves. This is accomplished by light to moderate circular digital pressure next to specific vertebra on the bladder meridian. Circular pressure is rythmic and synchronized with the (3) three phases of respiration: (a) holding breath (b) inhaling (c) exhaling.
    A word of caution here is necessary. To be effective the spinal vertebra need not be moved and indeed should not be moved by anyone who is not trained and licensed in this procedure. Should any problem arise from improper application of these techniques a licensed chiropractor should be consulted immediately.
    Extreme caution should be exercised with older people with severe osteoporosis, carcinoma, fractures of the spine, or patients who have been on prolonged cortisone therapy. Gentle accu-digipressure applied to the appropriate areas in unison with the proper breathing phases

## CHAPTER V: PREREQUISITES FOR A POSITIVE OUTCOME

will yield the desired result. With infants, just rubbing over the transverse processes (Figure 2 & 10) of the spinal segments while the baby laughs, giggles, cries or screams will do the trick. Muscle testing procedures for infants and very young children are done with an adult "stand in" or surrogate tester. This will be explained later in detail.

The photographs and diagrams in this book should prove sufficient to enable you to perform all procedures without difficulty. However, if you have lingering doubts or questions regarding the "How to", it is suggested that you acquire the instructional videotape which was expressly produced to demonstrate and clarify the primary techniques presented in this book. Seeing the techniques put into action makes it all seem quite easy.... which it really is! See Chapter XVI for more information.

# CHAPTER VI: APPLICATION OF THE TECHNIQUE

First we must decide whether the condition from which the patient suffers is indeed a cold. Other possibilities are allergies and flues.

To accomplish this we must learn simple muscle testing procedures. Proper testing is absolutely essential because it forms the basis upon which you will determine which bladder meridian points will be treated. Results will be no better than your ability to identify and reactivate short circuitry in the body.

The best time to apply "the cure" is when the cold victim is just "coming down" with a cold. That is to say when he feels the first chill, sneeze, or body ache. Often the cold can be stopped literally in it's tracks. This is the time to administer a sublingual dose of the homeopathic remedy Aconite 30X and Nux Vomica 30X. These can be obtained in a homeopathic pharmacy over the counter or from homeopathic suppliers. See Chapter XVI.

Give these remedies <u>after</u> the "Ten Minute Cure." A

dose of each five minutes apart should be sufficient. First Aconite 30X and five minutes later follow with a dose of Nux Vomica 30X. The other remedies listed in Chapter XII will be useful for certain symptomatic pictures but not essential to virus eradication.

## STEP ONE: TEST AN INTACT MUSCLE

This means to apply pressure against the patient's muscle resistance until it's a stalemate. You will feel a kind of "locking" sensation in the joint. This occurs at the relative neutralization point of opposing forces. When this joint lock "breaks" the patient can not sustain the muscle resistance. This indicates a positive test result. Although any intact muscle can be used, I prefer to use the anterior or medial deltoids for accessibility and convenience (Figures 6 & 7). If the muscle is strong "in the clear" it is suitable as a test indicator. "In the clear" means strong without having touched the body. If the anterior deltoid muscle is weak and falls toward the floor or table, turn the patient over and apply light to moderate accu-digipressure on the bladder meridian points next to the fourth dorsal (T4) vertebra (Figures 1,2 & 10) on each phase of respiration: a) Holding breath b) During inhalation c) During exhalation press and rub in a circular fashion. Retest the muscle. It should be strong. If not do again. If the medial deltoid is weak apply the correcting procedures described in chapter VIII relative to lung correction. Make sure you are next to the proper vertebra.

NOTE: The proper objective is to stimulate the nervous system where the nerves exit the spine as well as the sympathetic nerve ganglion which are located parallel to the spinal column (Figure 1). Avoid thrusting upon the spinal column. It is not necessary and may be detrimental to the patient and the curative process. Do not move the

## CHAPTER VI: APPLICATION OF THE TECHNIQUE

spinal vertebrae. Happily it is not required to obtain the desired results.

Muscle weakness may indicate gall bladder dysfunction or a shoulder injury. If initially weak and T4 corrective procedure makes it strong, the problem is usually the gall bladder and will be temporarily corrected by the procedure. If the shoulder is problematic use the other arm. If both are weak employ the hamstring muscle (Figure 8). If hamstrings are weak (Figures 1, 2 & 10) rub with moderate circular pressure briskly on the sacral base and the 5th lumbar bladder meridian points in respiratory phases. Rub hamstring muscular area. (Figure 2) This will usually make the muscle strong again. If not, employ a surrogate tester or use another intact muscle.

In contrast; an organ or gland may test strong in the clear when you contact a reflex point and test a muscle. This does not mean that the circuits are necessarily trouble free. Phase two and three testing procedures may reveal hidden weaknesses when applied.

Muscle testing is not a contest of strength between the healer and patient. One should use just enough force to test the integrity of the muscle and no more. Do not overpower your patient. It will only tire the muscle, ruin your indicator, and discourage the patient. You will, with practice, come to feel a familiar sensation when the joint locks. That is just the correct amount of pressure and resistance. When the muscle challenge goes to weakness the patient should not fight the process. Even pressure and resistance are essential each time a test is made. Consistency is the goal.

The next logical question is why we are doing all of this and what do we hope to accomplish? The answer is that by testing the integrity (strength) of the muscle we have a neurological standard against which to measure dysfunction. By touching a short circuit indicator (test point), a temporary interruption in the neural pathway renders the test muscle temporarily weak. If there is no problem in the circuitry the muscle remains strong.

FOR EXAMPLE: If the test muscle is strong and we touch the cold test point and the muscle goes weak, we get immediate confirmation that the patient has a cold and is in need of the "Ten Minute Cure" (Figure 12). If the test point tests strong, the patient may still have a cold but may require additional testing and correction to "surface" the condition — which leads us to step two.

## STEP TWO: ISOLATE THE PROBLEM & ACTIVATE BIO-COMPUTER

On a strip of blotter paper write the words clearly "Your Cold Virus." Next, stick it under the patient's tongue and soak it with saliva (remember to keep the written impression dry). Next take a sample of nasal secretions on a cotton swab. Viruses are heavily concentrated in nasal secretion. Put the swab and the blotter paper in a plastic bag. Wash your hands. Washing hands frequently among members of large families will help to reduce the contagious factor where the cold gets passed from one to the other and back again. Now as the patient inhales ask him to grasp the plastic bag in the left hand. What this does is to access the bio-computer by reintroducing the toxic substance into the biosphere or auric field. The in-breath is symbolic of input to the bio-computer. By using the saliva, nose swabs, and written vibrational component we cover all bases. This collection of toxic material is referred to as a "witness."

The muscle is tested against the biological input. A weakness indicates confirmation of the question. The patient is infected with cold virus. If you have physically overpowered the individual or have mentally concepted

## CHAPTER VI: APPLICATION OF THE TECHNIQUE

a preconceived notion you will get a false reading. This is why you must keep an open mind. The patient's symptom picture may lead you to draw a hasty conclusion as to a causative agent. You must activate the bio-computer in a sequential manner to effect a cure. Take nothing for granted. Approach this step by step, line upon line. Additionally you must focus on the desire to know the patient's condition and mentally rule out any possibility of reflecting your own internal weakness or infection. This is done simply with will and intent by mentally setting these parameters at the outset.

For further confirmation, test the cold point and challenge the muscle — strength indicates a cold virus infection and activates the bio-computer to accept the cure sequence. This procedure works on the great majority of people and you can proceed with the subsequent steps as outlined.

NOTE: In the presence of the "witness" which gives muscle weakness, when a cold is present, touching the cold point will make the muscle test strong. Without a witness, weakness is a positive confirmation when the cold point alone is contacted. Use one test to confirm the other.

In rare cases one must be more specific and name the specific virus or condition. <u>FOR EXAMPLE:</u> 1. "Your Rhinovirus" (sneezing, head cold, runny nose); 2. "Your Adenovirus" (chest cold/sore throat, red drippy eyes); 3. "Your Corona Virus" (dull ache, rotton feeling); 4. "Your Cold Syndrome" (the whole nine yards); 5. "Your Cold Virus Toxins" (do after "Your Cold Virus"). You may have to run these additional patterns even after you have fixed "Your Cold Virus." In some highly sensitive individuals you may need to use: 6. "Your Histamine Reaction." If any of these witnesses test weak, apply the following identical procedures. <u>"The condition or</u>

## CHAPTER VI: APPLICATION OF THE TECHNIQUE

<u>symptom may appear to be different but the principle for cure remains ever the same."</u> Be flexible and be creative! <u>Exception</u>: If after proper preparation of the witness you get no response (weakness) to the witness or the cold test point perform the testing and correction procedures described in Chapter VIII for sore throats.

The clearing of the throat reflex will "unmask" the condition and open up the body's circuitry to permit the witness to perform its' normal function. This type of problem does not often occur but must be kept in mind.

### STEP THREE: <u>NORMALIZE LIVER FUNCTION</u>

Once your body has identified the condition to be treated (common cold) indicated by test muscle weakness in the presence of the witness, put your free hand on the liver reflex area (Figure 9). The muscle will get strong indicating that liver function has been interfered with and must be corrected. Patient does not hold the liver reflex area while corrections are made in phase I. Turn the patient over on his stomach. Using the thumbs in rythmic circular fashion apply accu-digipressure to the bladder meridian points of the 2nd dorsal, 5th dorsal, and 8th dorsal segments on the three phases of respiration (Figures 2 & 10).

This is a phase one correction.

Remember, there is no need to be rough or use excessive pressure. A gentle to moderate intermittent pressure will do the job of reintergrating the circuitry and ousting the virus. Practice until you have mastered the precise amount of force to apply. Your technique should cause minimal or no discomfort to the patient, yet must be sufficient to make the correction. This will be made

# CHAPTER VI: APPLICATION OF THE TECHNIQUE

known by a strong muscle indicator following the correction. Retest the hamstring muscle against the reflex point; it will be strong. If not strong you either did the correction improperly or the hamstring is weak in the clear. Weak in the "clear" means the muscle tests weak without your having touched any reflex points or spinal segments.

NOTE: weakness of the hamstring muscle in the clear has nothing to do with the cold virus procedure and will give you a false impression. Make sure the hamstring is intact before continuing.

To check the hamstring first take the witness from the patient and place him on his stomach as demonstrated (Figure 8). If it tests weak in the clear, rub briskly on the sacral base and 5th lumbar bladder meridian points on the (3) phases of respiration and rub the additional indicated points briskly (Figures 1, 2 & 10). Now the muscle should test strong. If not, sit the patient up and use the deltoid muscle group for a test indicator (Figures 6 & 7).

Reintroduce the witness to the patient in the prescribed manner before continuing.

If you have previously tested the hamstring and are sure of its integrity there is no need to withdraw and reintroduce the witness once initiated.

Now have the patient hold his liver with his primary hand and the witness with the other. Starting with the 1st cervical vertebra touch each vertebra individually with your free hand (fingertips) testing against the hamstring or deltoid muscle for strength or weakness. Each segment that tests weak must be stimulated via the bladder meridian points. Work your way down the spine from top to bottom.

Each vertebra that goes weak should be corrected by bladder meridian point pressure in the prescribed manner until all test strong. Do this from $C_1$ to the coccyx. Do not apply pressure directly on the coccyx or tip of the tail bone if it tests weak; rather rub with moderate digital pressure on the marked bladder meridian points parallel to the coccyx (Figures 1 & 2). They will most likely be sore. Retest for strength.

This completes a phase two correction.

When all vertebral circuits test strong, instruct the patient to join the thumb and pinky finger on both hands in a circular configuration (Figure 11). Hold the witness with one hand and touch the liver with the other making sure the thumb pinky are joined. Test each vertebra from the coccyx to the 1st cervical. This configuration introduces additional circuits. Test each spinal segment from bottom to top. Correct bladder meridian points adjacent to each segment that tests weak until all test strong. This is a phase three correction. Break the thumb/pinky configuration and do step IV.

Remember not to overtire the muscle. Switch legs or arms as necessary. If true weakness is not demonstrated stimulation is not required. Check each test point with the patient's hand open and in thumb/pinky configuration. You may find weakness in one or more phases. Fix what you find. Check from top to bottom with the patient's hand open, and from bottom to top in thumb/pinky configuration (circuits A & B).

## STEP FOUR: NORMALIZE THYMUS & SPLEEN FUNCTION

To normalize the thymus and spleen function, first withdraw the witness from the patient. Touch the thymus test point and challenge the muscle indicator (Figures 12 & 12.1). If weak turn the patient on his stomach or sit him up and correct the bladder meridian points adjacent to the

9th dorsal vertebra. This is a phase one correction. If done correctly the muscle will be strong. Now have the patient contact the thymus point and hold it while testing and correction is made. Identify any additional weak vertebral segments and correct exactly as outlined in Step III. The only difference is that the thymus point is held instead of the liver. This is a phase two correction. Then, put the patient into thumb/pinky configuration and complete phase three correction procedure. Reflex points are held while corrections are made in phase II & III only.

Next repeat the same procedure with the spleen (Figure 13 & 13.1). If the spleen demonstrates weakness stimulate the bladder meridian points adjacent to $T_1$, $T_5$, $T_9$. This is a phase one correction. Then have the patient hold the spleen test point. Test and stimulate bladder meridian points opposite each weak segment until all test strong on both A and B circuits (open hand/thumb-pinky). All three phase corrections are required.

NOTE: If the thymus or spleen points are strong when initially contacted, omit the phase one procedure and proceed to phases two and three. Make any corrections as indicated. Check thymus/spleen or spleen/thymus in reverse order. Proper sequence is often a factor in total reintergration of circuitry. This means if you do not get weakness upon phase one testing of the thymus, you may get it testing the spleen. After fixing the spleen points retest the thymus; it may then demonstrate weakness.

## STEP FIVE: CORRECT COLD AND SINUS POINTS

At this point the witness is still withdrawn from the patient. The action of holding a reflex point becomes a localized witness for specific treatment procedure. Retest the cold test point (Figures 14 & 14.1). If weak, dig your thumb into it and do a deep circular massage. It will hurt a little but rub it until the point tests strong. Do both hand points separately, testing each separately. Next test the sinus points touching them (Figures 15 and 15.1) with your fingertips. Test them altogether or one at a time; if weak massage each in a circular manner until all test strong. This is a phase one point correction.

Additional phase corrections are not required, unless points will not correct by digital stimulation. In this event hold the points and check liver/thymus/spleen reflex points individually. If by touching any one of these points the muscle indicator becomes strong, have the patient hold sinus points with one hand and the appropriate organ reflex point with the other. Use the hamstring muscle for a test indicator and apply phase one, two and/ or three correction techniques specific to the organ in question (see steps III and IV). If no reflex point can be found to strengthen the muscle, have the patient hold the points as you check each vertebra individually from top to bottom in phase two and bottom to top in phase three.

In this instance you will fix those vertebral levels that make the muscle indicator strong. This is necessary because your test muscle is weak while holding the points.

After correcting all strong segmental indicators via bladder meridian accu-digipressure, break and reestablish point contact. This time retest and correct any segmental indicators that perpetuate weakness. Retest the reflex points; they will be strong. This constitutes phase II & III point correction procedures. You will rarely have to go this far to obtain correction.

### STEP SIX: STIMULATE BODY'S NATURAL ANTIBIOTIC POINT

Traditional oriental medicine states that the accupuncture point at end of the cubital crease in the folded arm at

# CHAPTER VI: APPLICATION OF THE TECHNIQUE

the elbow stimulates the body's ability to create a natural antibiotic effect. While difficult to prove empirically, clinical experience has shown these points to be active in many cold cases. Treatment of these points seems to be efficacious in warding off opportunistic bacterial infections that sometimes hitchhike a ride with viral invaders and take advantage of a stressed immune system. Locate the point (Figure 5) with your index or middle finger. This becomes your witness. Test an intact muscle. If the muscle tests weak massage the point in a circular fashion with moderate digital pressure until the muscle tests strong. This is a phase one point correction. If the muscle tests strong on initial contact, then no stimulation is required. If positive the point is usually quite sore to the touch.

Although additional phase testing is usually not necessary it can be employed to enhance the effect. If this is desired, have the patient hold the point which now tests strong either before or after stimulation and employ phase two and three techniques. Fix any weaknesses you find.

If weak and digital point stimulation is ineffective perform your phase two and/or three correction by having the patient hold the points and find and fix the bladder meridian points adjacent to vertebra(e) which demonstrate strength. Then break and reestablish point contact and proceed with phase correction procedures fixing only those vertebral levels that perpetuate weakness. The procedures are identical to those outlined in Step V.

<u>One final note of importance:</u>

If testing in the clear for any step in this procedure demonstrates no weakness, yet the patient shows obvious symptoms, go directly to phase two and three challange and corrective procedures. This will surface the condition so the body can deal with it. Make no corrections by stimulation of bladder meridian points in the absence of positive indicators. Do not create problems where they do not exist! The old mechanic's adage "If it works don't fix it," is based upon wise practical experience.

Now reintroduce the witness to the patient. Retest circuits A and B in the clear. If weak on either, recheck your work. If strong on both, this concludes the phase correction procedures for the Ten Minute Cure. If chest symptoms (cough) or sore throat is present refer to chapter VIII for corrective procedures before retesting the witness.

### STEP SEVEN: <u>NORMALIZE BODY Ph FACTOR</u>

To get the body Ph factor back to the alkaline side, which seems to be antithetical to cold virus activity, encourage the patient to take a double dose of effervescent antacid. This is not for those with heart problems. Children should not be given a variety of antacid with aspirin. People with aspirin allergy should consume the non-aspirin variety. This is optional and not a necessity to rid the body of the cold virus. It does, however, discourage reinfection.

Lack of tissue oxygenation is a prime factor in illness. Acidic conditions rob the tissues of available oxygen and hamper the recovery process. Viruses and many other micro-organisms evolved at a time in history when oxygen was not as plentiful as it is today: that is why they thrive while we suffer. Greedy commercial interests have raped our rain forests and polluted our oceans. Trees and the once plentiful ocean algae are our main sources of oxygen. Without adequate oxygen levels on the planet man cannot hope to maintain proper health. Until sanctions and fines exceed the cost of cleaning up our planet, it is unlikely that industry will cooperate. We need to focus on survival issues not on the "Bottom Line" of corporate financial statements.

## CONGRATULATIONS! YOU HAVE JUST GIVEN THE COLD VIRUS THE OLD "HEAVE HO!"

After treatment the patient should partake of light nourishment, plenty of fluids, and get adequate rest. This gives the immune system time to recuperate.

Once the technique is mastered the cure need not take more than 10 minutes. You have only assisted the immune system in ousting the unwanted invader, not conferred lasting immunity. If the individual's immune system and general condition is at a low ebb, you may have to repeat the procedure later the same day or the following day. All circuits must be cleared and reactivated. Failure to do so may result in the virus regaining a foothold or reinfection by another virus. The more proficient you become in practice the less likely this becomes.

Keep in mind that all people are different and their symptoms and patterns will vary according to many unseen factors. Look past this confusing complexity to the end result. Stick to the technique with conviction. The natural inclination of the body to heal will do the rest.

Proper diet, keeping the colon clean and super oxygenation of the body systems are the mainstays of immunity. Oxygenation of the body may be assisted by the use of organic Germanium 132 in combination with co-enzyme Q. A less expensive method is to add two (2) drops of food grade hydrogen peroxide ($H_2O_2$) to eight (8) onces of filtered drinking water. The FDA long ago approved the use of hydrogen peroxide as an additive to milk for long life shelf packaging.

When $H_2O_2$ gives up an oxygen atom, that atom

oxidizes lipid envelope viruses and many other disease organisms as well without harming normal blood cells. Hydrogen peroxide should never be used unless diluted to levels not exceeding $1/2$ of one percent or less. A standard bath tub full of water with 1 - 6 pints of store variety $H_2O_2$ will allow the patient to absorb this benefit directly through the skin.

WARNING:

Ingestion of standard 3 or 35% hydrogen peroxide solution <u>undiluted</u> kills! Drugstore variety 3% $H_2O_2$, which is not as pure as food-grade hydrogen peroxide, should not be taken internally. The following dilution factor can be considered safety therapeutic:

35% strength = 2 drops/8oz. glass of filtered water.

The 3% solution is to be used to gargle, make a bath solution or brush the teeth. It is a superior external disinfectant. Gargle: 1 part 3% $H_2O_2$ to 3 parts water is the recommended effective dilution factor. This will also be beneficial for infected gum conditions as well as septic sore throat.

The tooth brush becomes a dangerous agent for reinfection during illness. Rinse the bristles thoroughly after brushing with 3% hydrogen peroxide to prevent recontaminating yourself the next time you brush.

Always muscle test to see if dose or therapy is acceptable to the body. This procedure is helpful in maintaining good health but do not expect it to be a "cure-all".

# INSTRUCTIONAL
# DIAGRAMS
# and
# PHOTOGRAPHS

# CHAPTER VI: APPLICATION OF THE TECHNIQUE

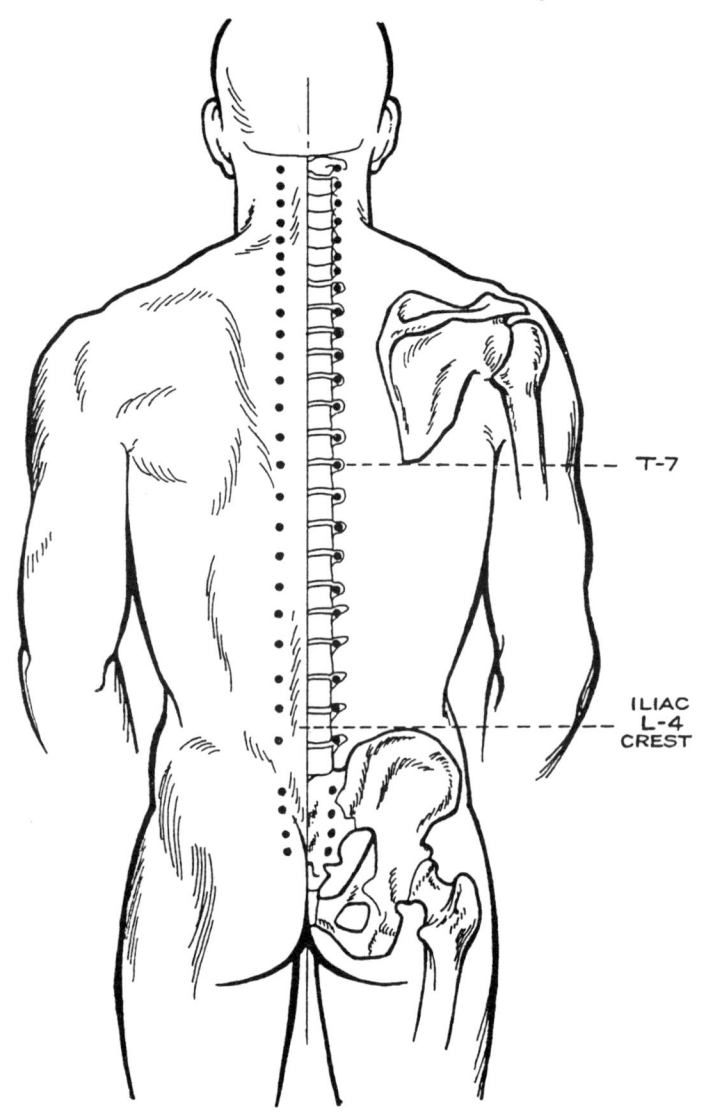

Fig. 1   Bladder Meridian and Accu-digipressure Points.

# CHAPTER VI: APPLICATION OF THE TECHNIQUE

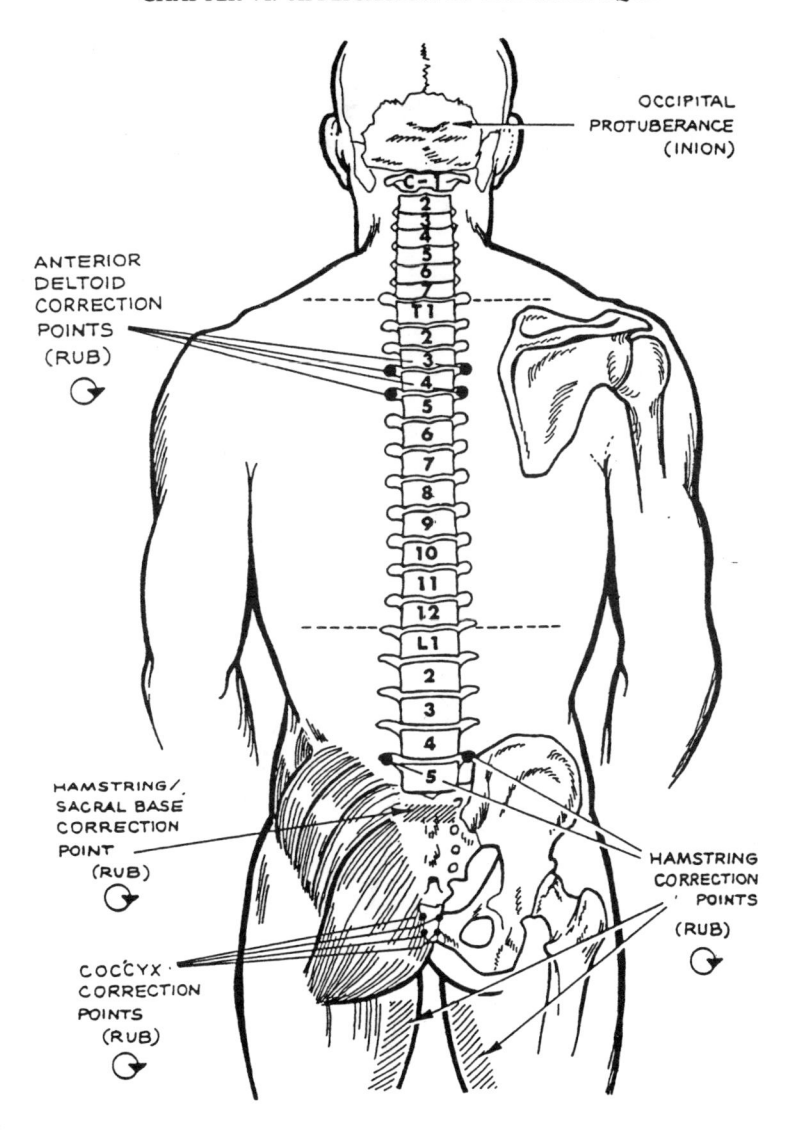

Fig. 2  Diagram of the spinal column, anterior deltoid/hamstring muscle/sacral base, coccyx correction points.

# CHAPTER VI: APPLICATION OF THE TECHNIQUE

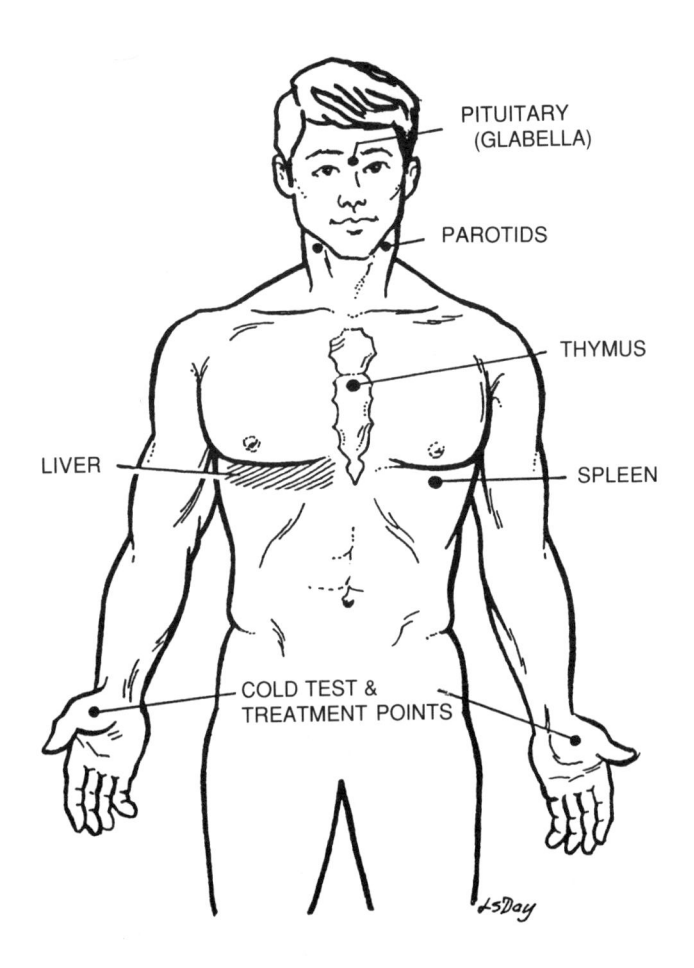

Fig. 3  Cold, liver, thymus, spleen, pituitary, throat (parotid glands) test and reflex points.

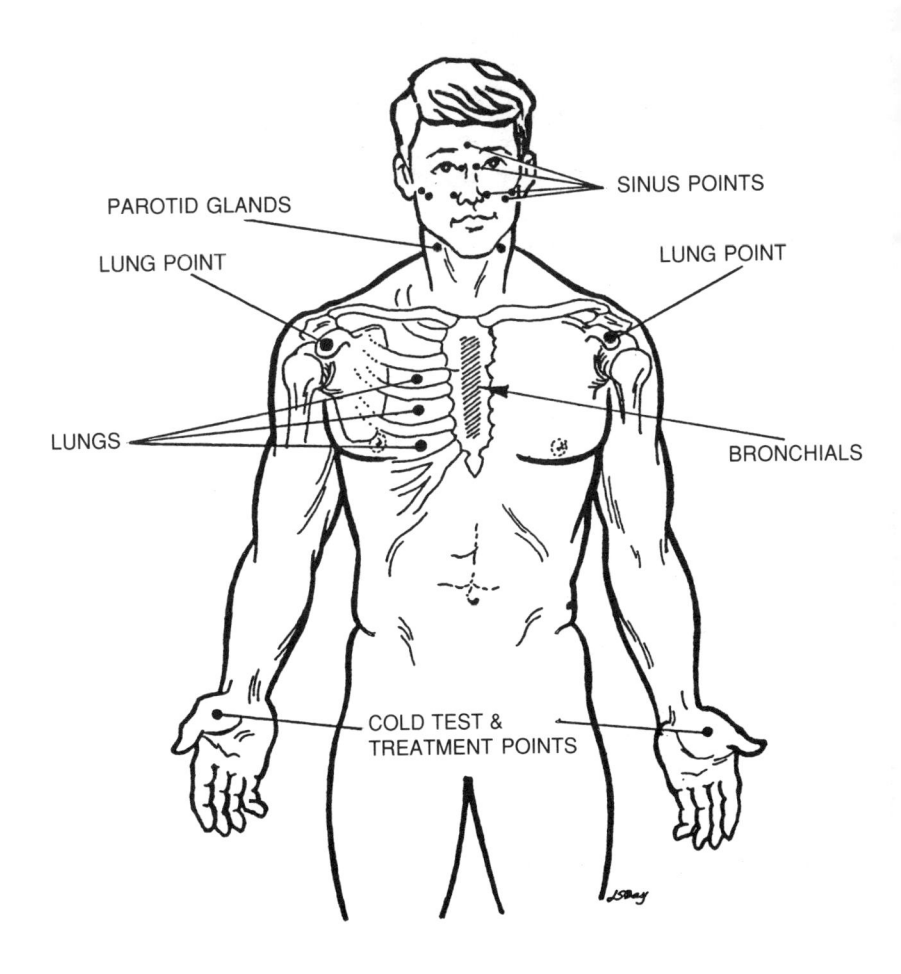

Fig. 4  Cold, sinus, lung, bronchial reflex points.

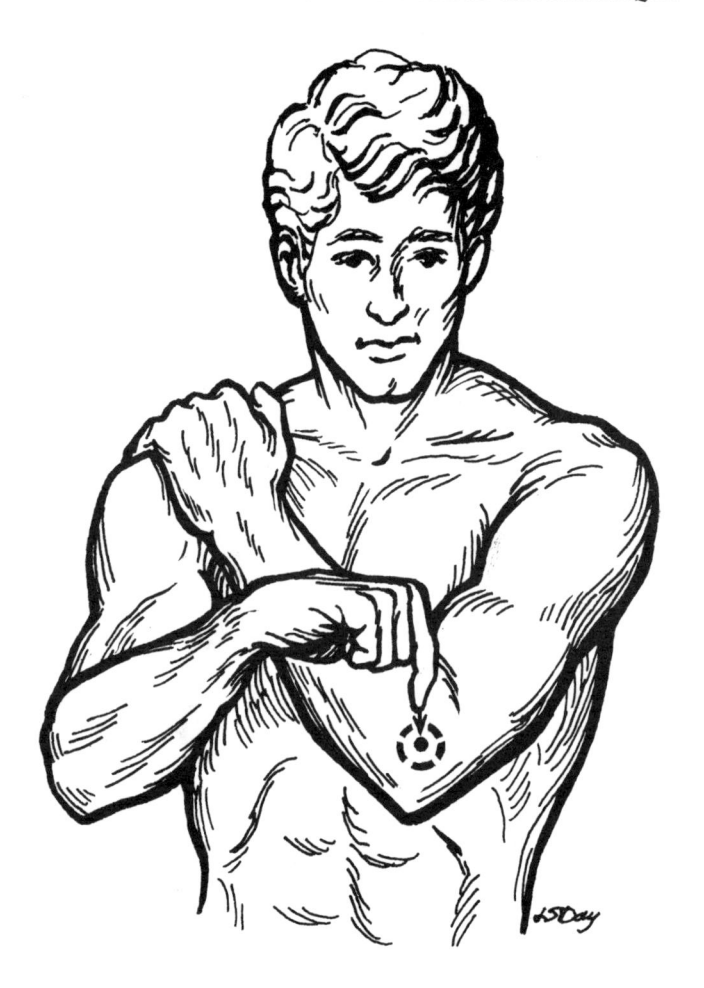

Fig. 5    Testing body's natural antibiotic stimulation point.

CHAPTER VI: APPLICATION OF THE TECHNIQUE      47

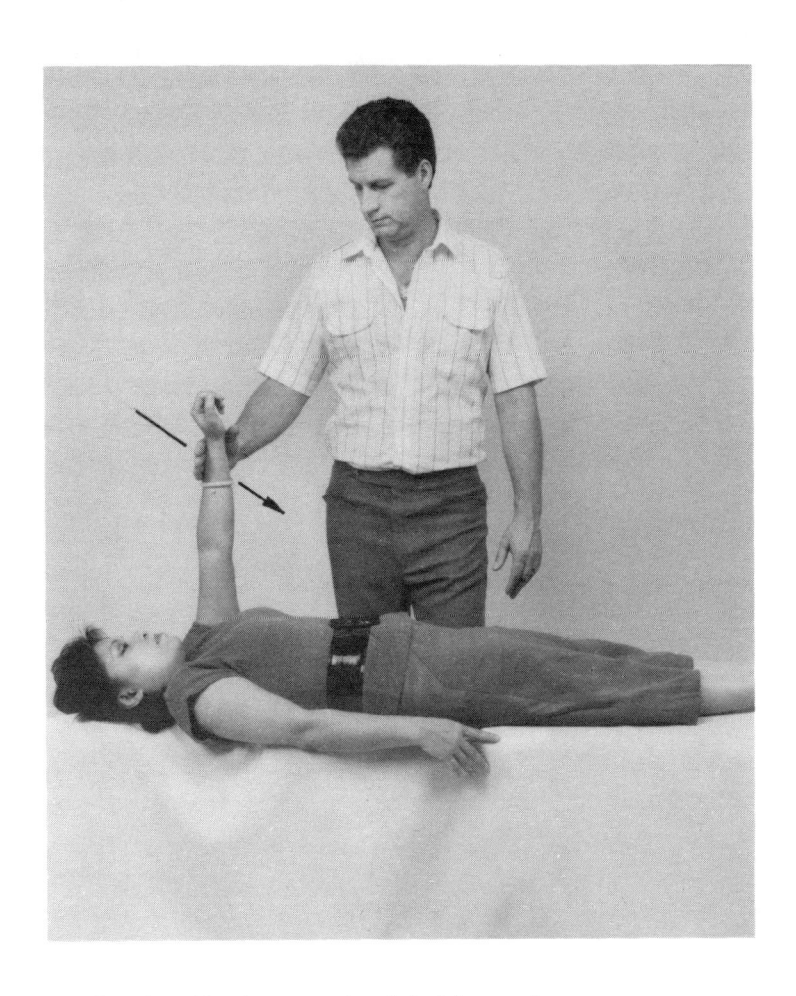

Fig. 6     Testing anterior deltoid muscle.

48　　　　CHAPTER VI: APPLICATION OF THE TECHNIQUE

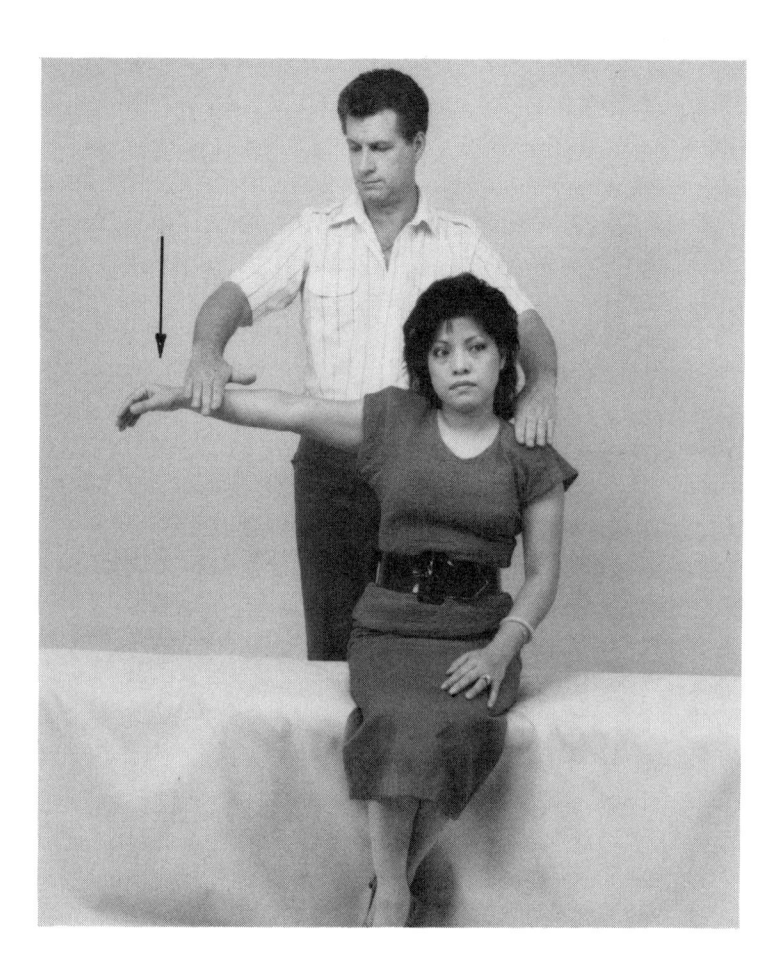

Fig. 7　　Testing medial deltoid muscle.

# CHAPTER VI: APPLICATION OF THE TECHNIQUE

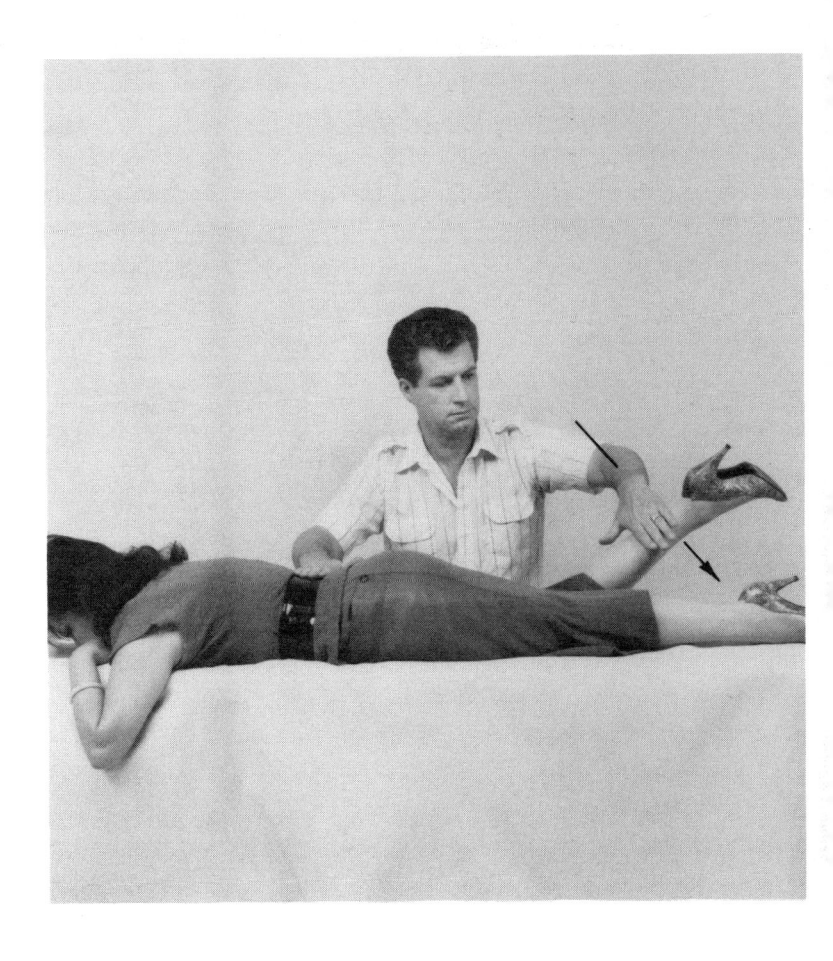

Fig. 8  Testing hamstring muscle.

50 CHAPTER VI: APPLICATION OF THE TECHNIQUE

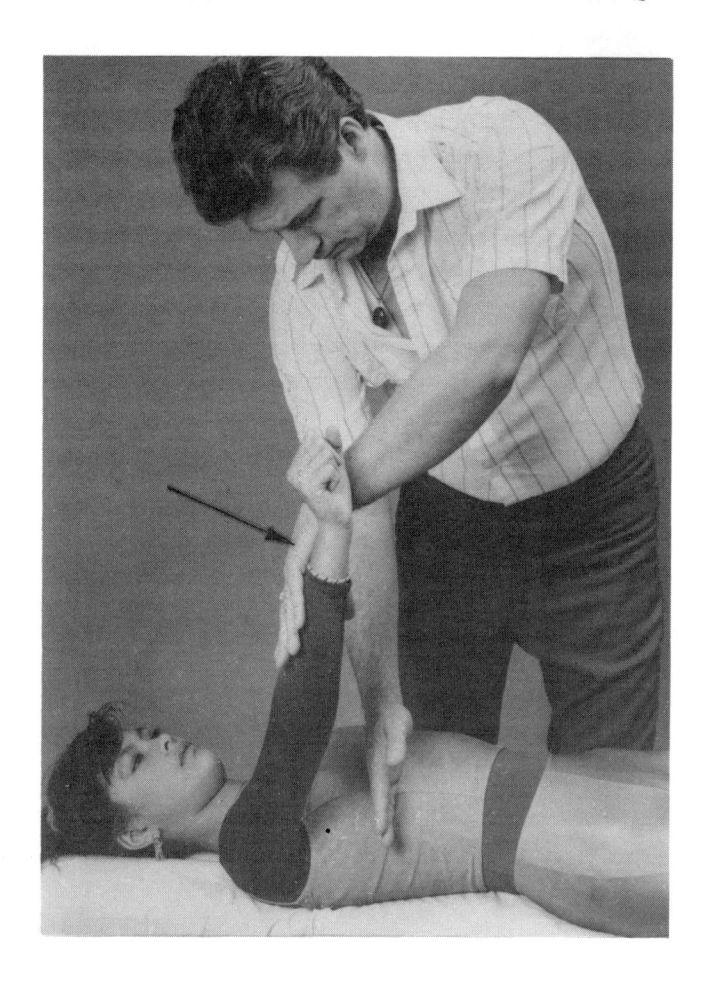

Fig. 9   Testing liver reflex area.

CHAPTER VI: APPLICATION OF THE TECHNIQUE 51

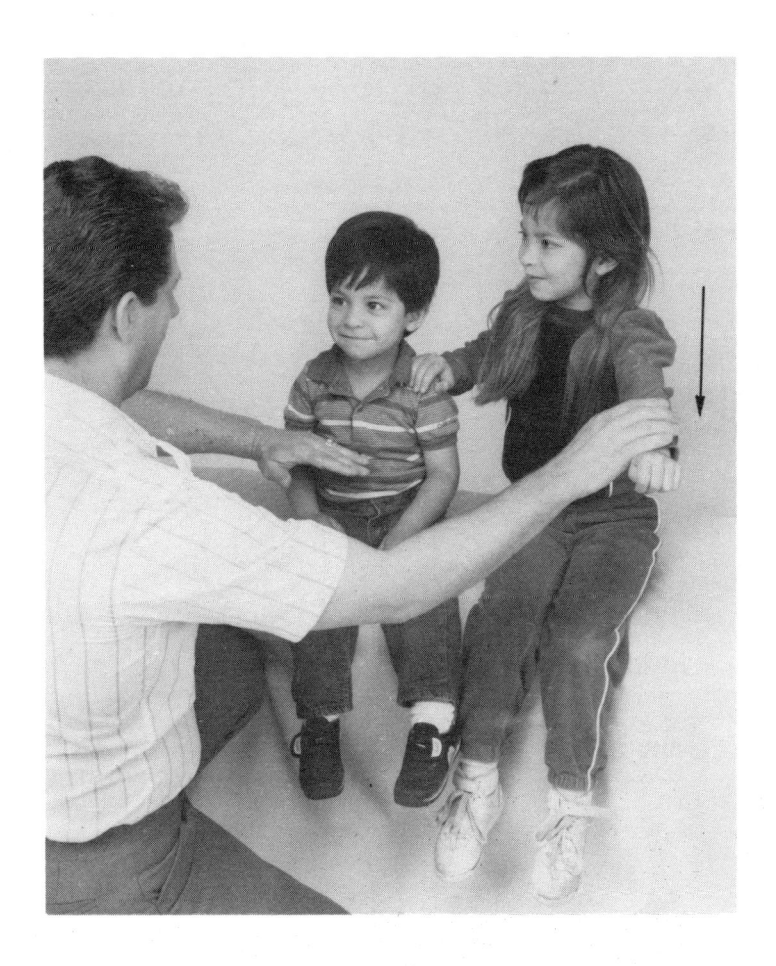

Fig. 9.1   Testing liver reflex area with surrogate.

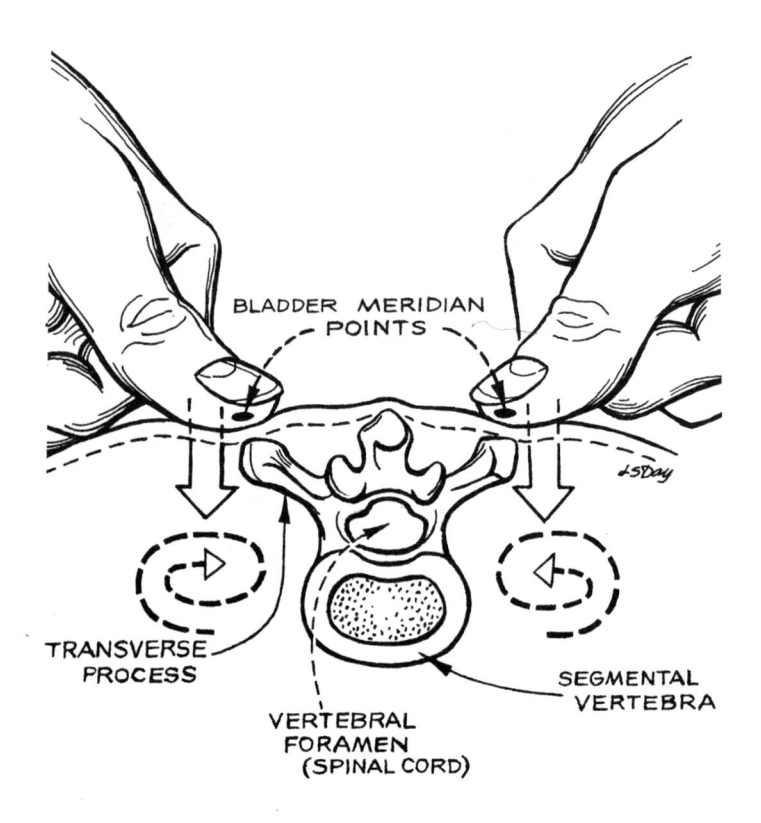

Fig. 10  Contacting bladder meridian points.

CHAPTER VI: APPLICATION OF THE TECHNIQUE 53

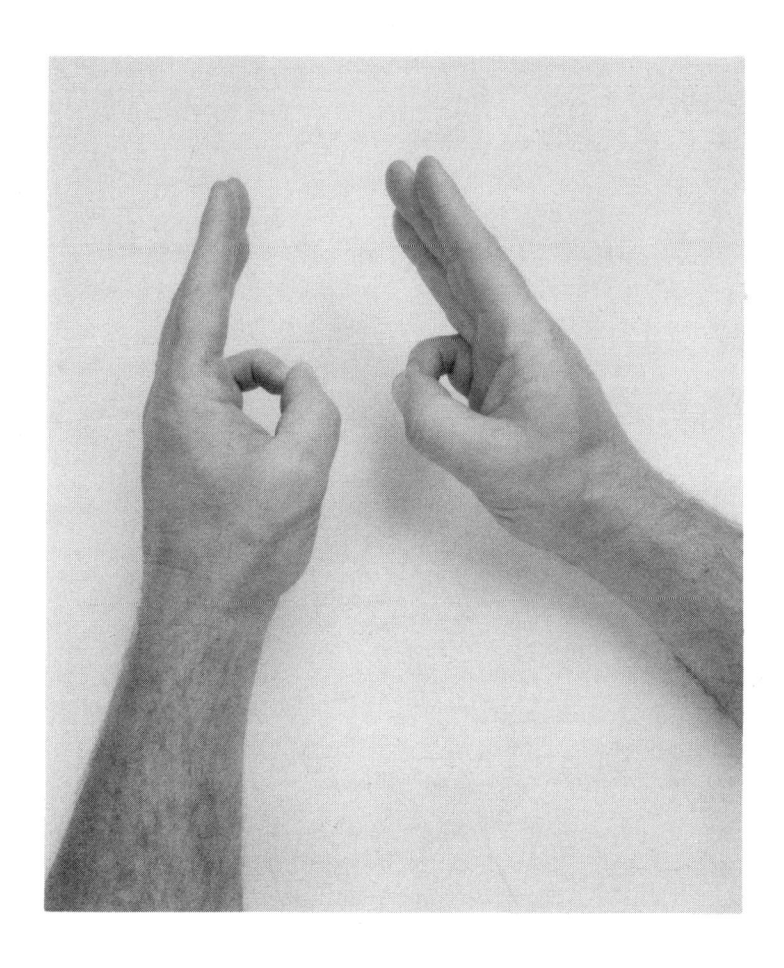

Fig. 11   Thumb/pinky configuration.

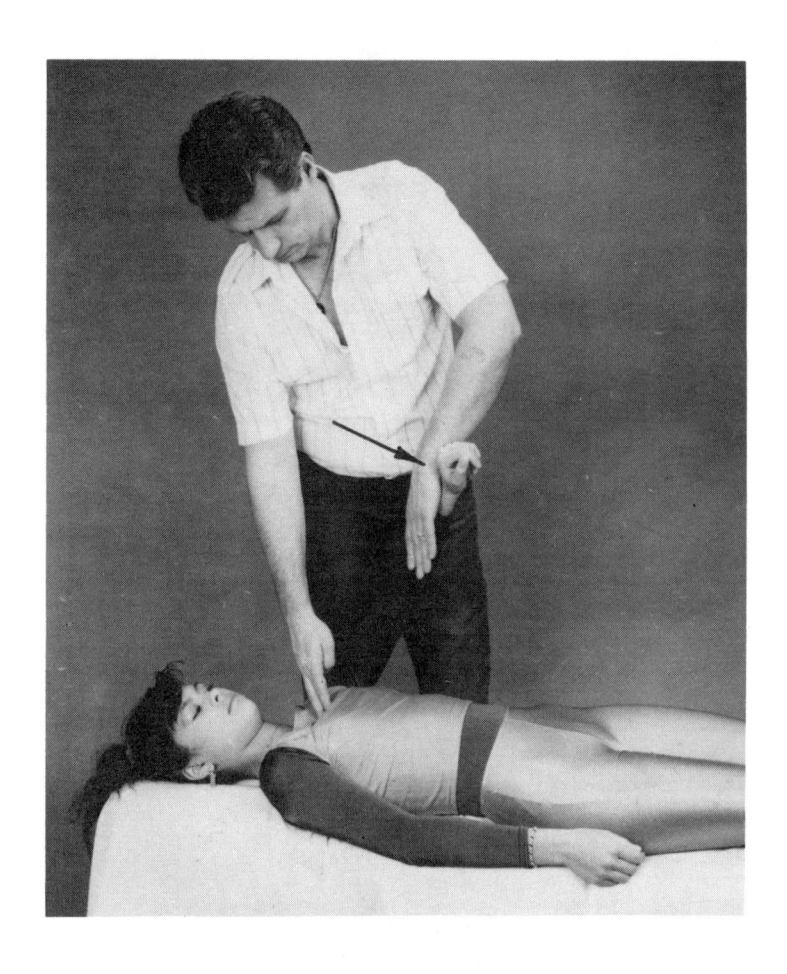

Fig. 12   Testing thymus reflex point.

CHAPTER VI: APPLICATION OF THE TECHNIQUE 55

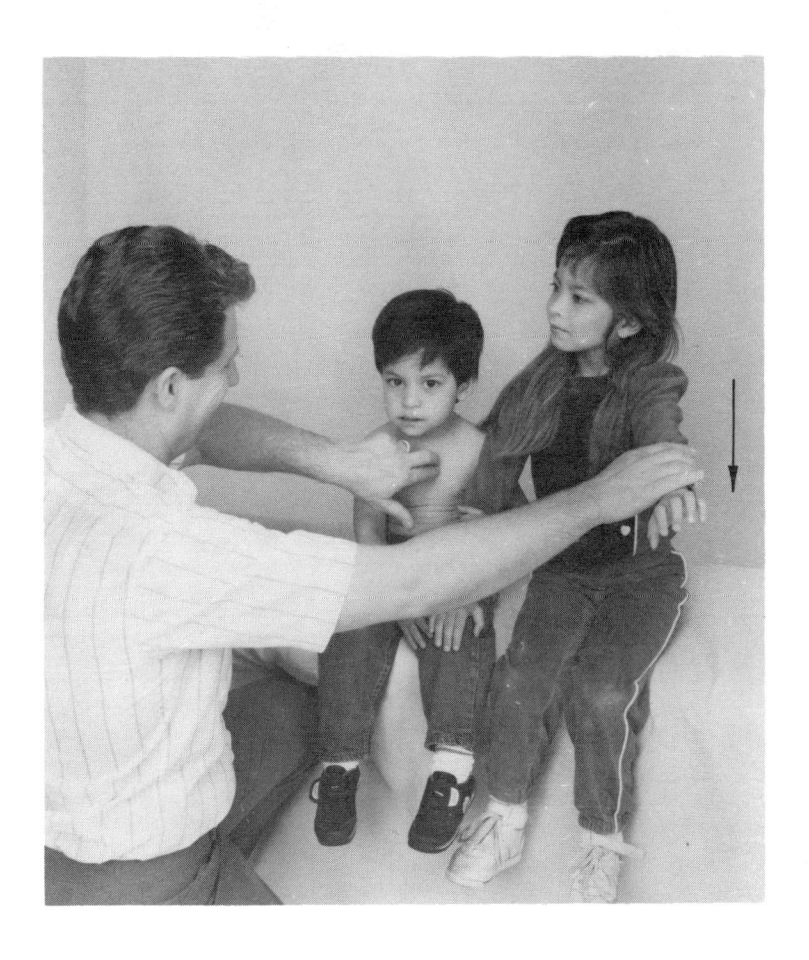

Fig. 12.1 Testing thymus reflex point with surrogate.

# CHAPTER VI: APPLICATION OF THE TECHNIQUE

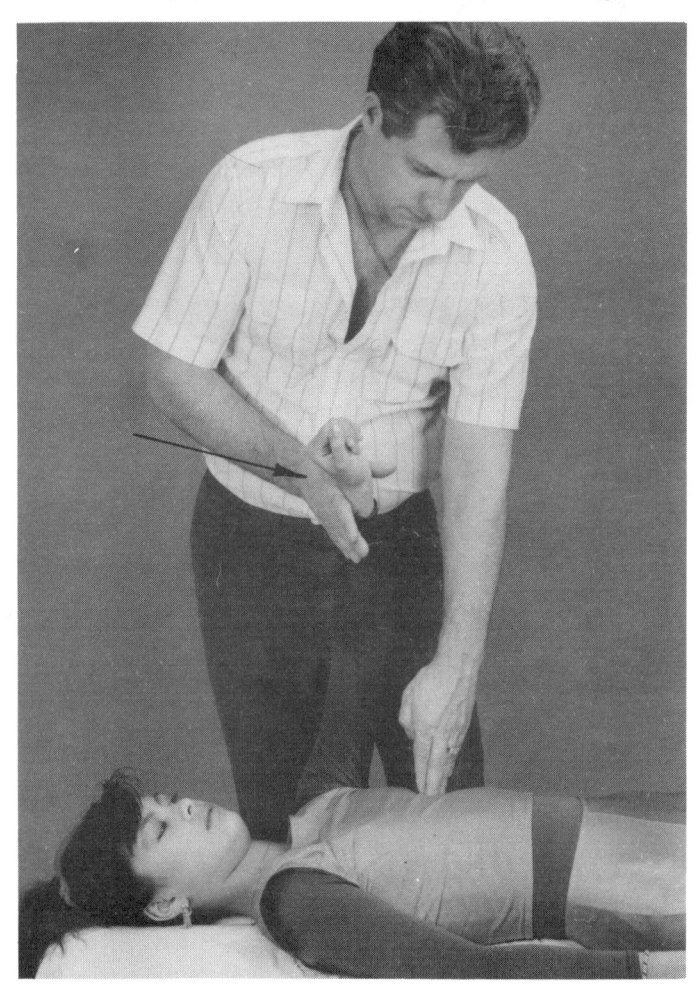

Fig. 13   Testing spleen reflex point.

# CHAPTER VI: APPLICATION OF THE TECHNIQUE

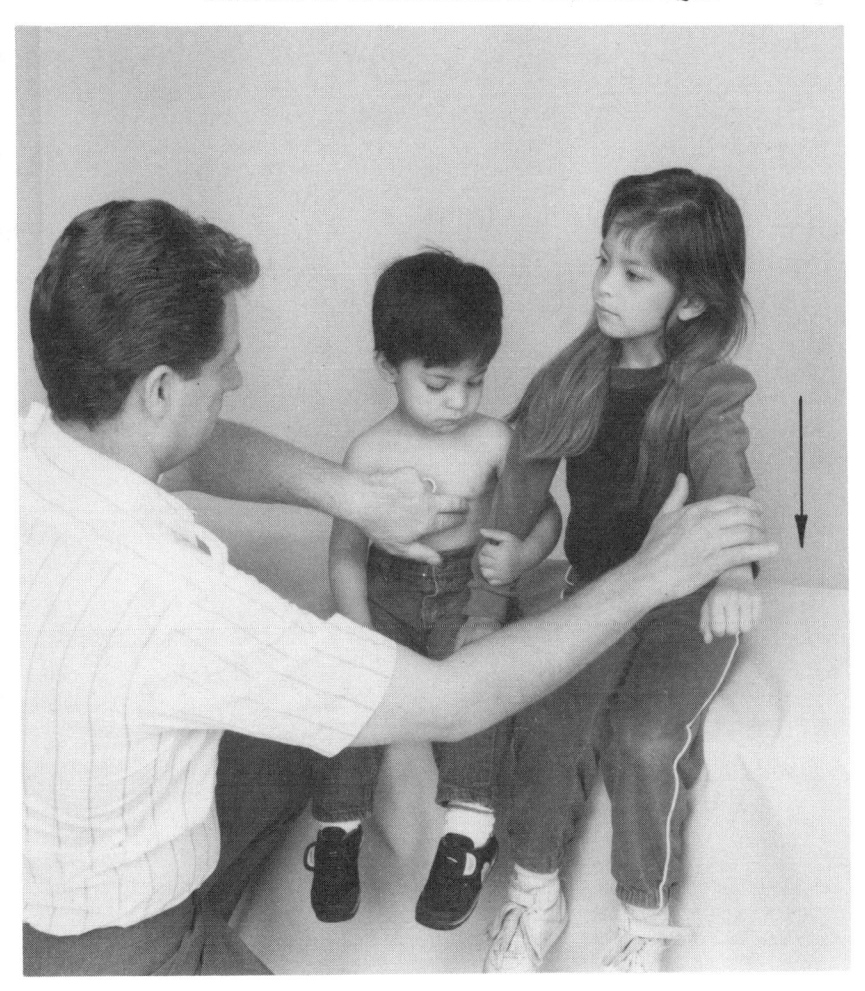

Fig. 13.1  Testing spleen reflex point with surrogate.

# CHAPTER VI: APPLICATION OF THE TECHNIQUE

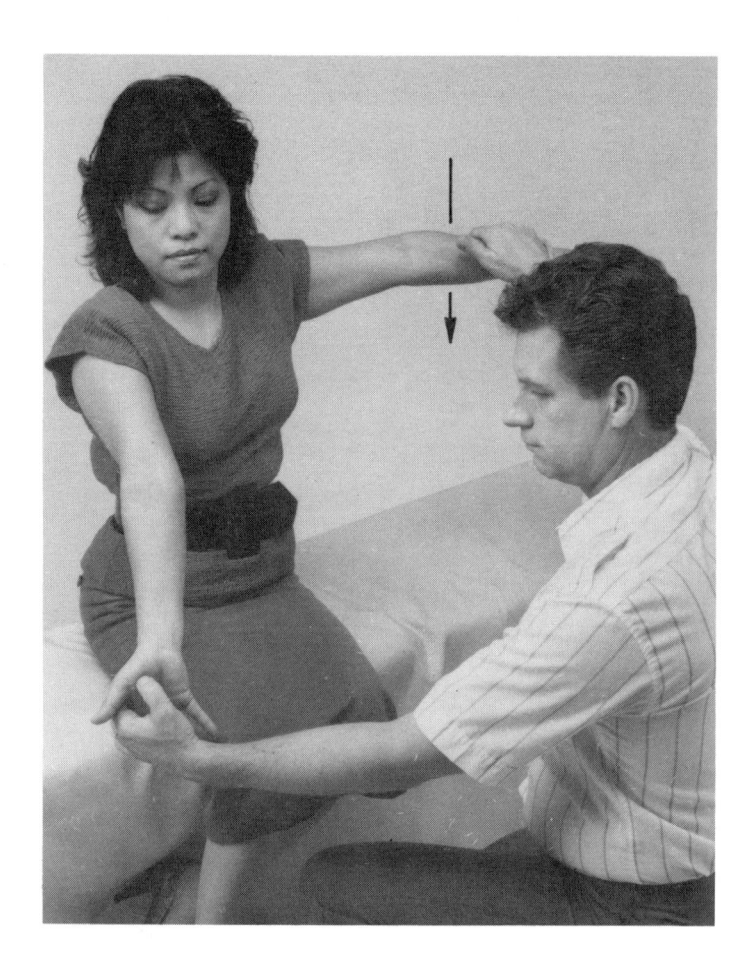

Fig. 14   Testing cold test and treatment point.

# CHAPTER VI: APPLICATION OF THE TECHNIQUE

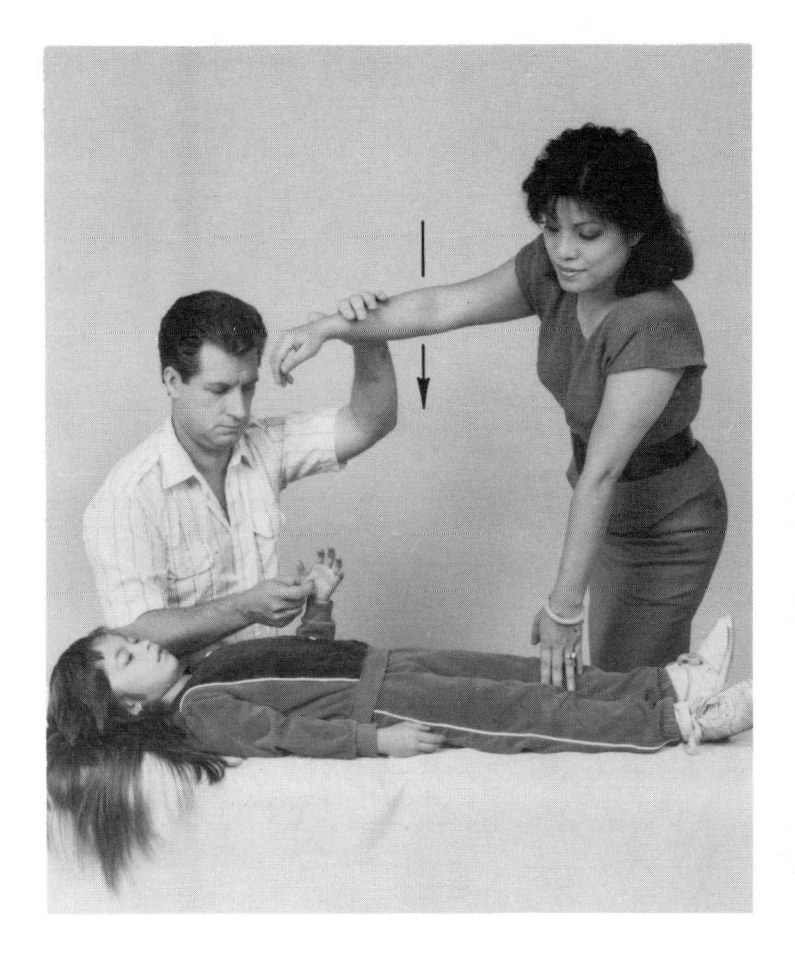

Fig. 14.1 Testing cold test and treatment point with surrogate.

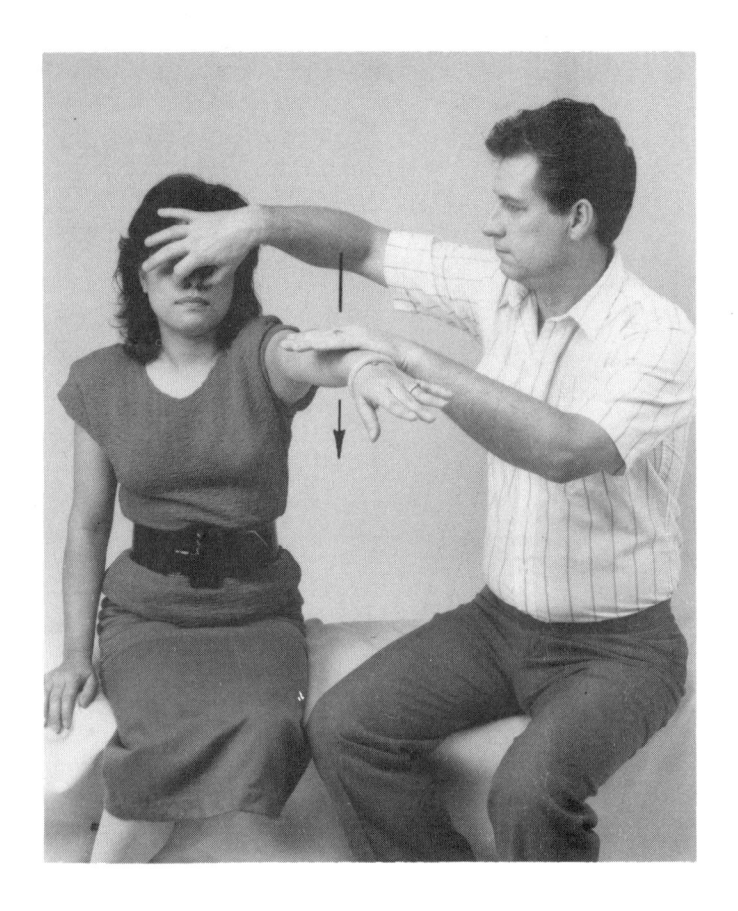

Fig. 15    Testing sinus reflex points.

# CHAPTER VI: APPLICATION OF THE TECHNIQUE 61

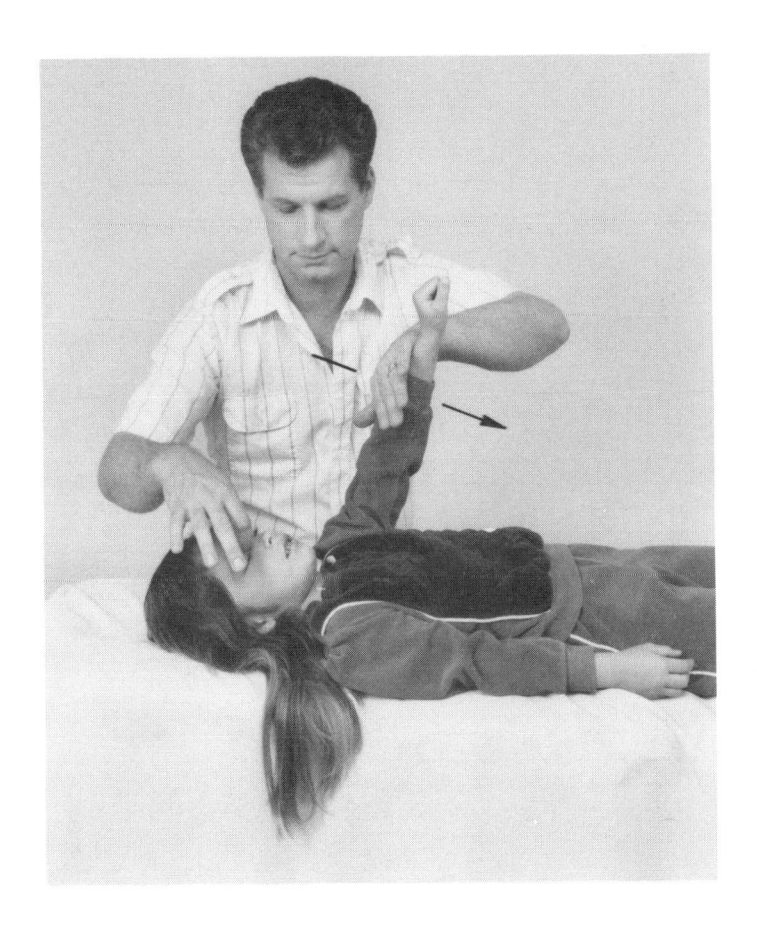

Fig. 15.1 Testing sinus reflex points.

# CHAPTER VII:
# TESTING PROCEDURES FOR THE HANDICAPPED, BEDRIDDEN, YOUNG CHILDREN, AND INFANTS

You will be happy to know that the procedures are identical with the exception of testing the biological circuitry. In these cases a "stand in" or surrogate tester is employed. The "stand in" will act as an electromagnetic shunt for the patient's energies. By testing the surrogate you will be able to assess and treat the patient.

How is this possible? The answer is again to be found in the process of mental agreement. When all three agree on the desired goal, that is what manifests. The Bible reminds us of this principle when the Master said, "when 2 or 3 are gathered in my name I shall be among them." The "I" referred to is the Christ, Higher Self or Inner Physician, to whichever term you may wish to relate. It is through this force or agency that true healing comes. The bottom line is that the surrogate principle works!

STEPS TO FOLLOW

The position of the patient is not crucial in this instance. First, test the surrogate's muscle integrity (Figures 16 & 17). If inadequate fix it or use another muscle. Be sure surrogates are not ill themselves. For babies I prefer to use the mother or true father because of the strong genetic connection. If not available anyone will do. The surrogate will not enter into the transaction in any way save to pass along the required information.

With one hand the surrogate touches any convenient part of the patient's body. This establishes contact. The other arm will be used as the test indicator. Apply Steps I-VI with the aid of the surrogate (Figures 9.1, 12.1, 13.1 & 14.1). Make the appropriate corrections using the surrogate for confirmation. For babies, the very elderly or infirm patients use only light to moderate digital pressure over the transverse processes of specific vertebra on the bladder meridian points. Make no effort to move any bones. Rub with intermittent pressure in a circular motion as the patient breathes. Et Voila! Do not make this a complicated affair. All you've done is use an extension handle to make your work easier. This principle applies equally to remedy testing as well.

POINTS TO REMEMBER

The condition must be identified, individual circuits challenged and assessed before curative input will be accepted and processed. When this is done systematically, processing and correction is instantaneous. Some people respond better to muscle testing techniques than others. For a surrogate choose the best candidate; experience will be your teacher. If the patient or surrogate is stronger than you, reduce the angle of the arm or leg so you have more leverage (Figure 17). The principle of joint lock still applies. The practitioner and patient should strive to keep both challenge and resistance to challenge consistently equal, without straining the muscle. If the patient does not have the knack for it, employ a surrogate. Don't swim against the current. Results are proportionate to the ability to properly assess and correct the problem.

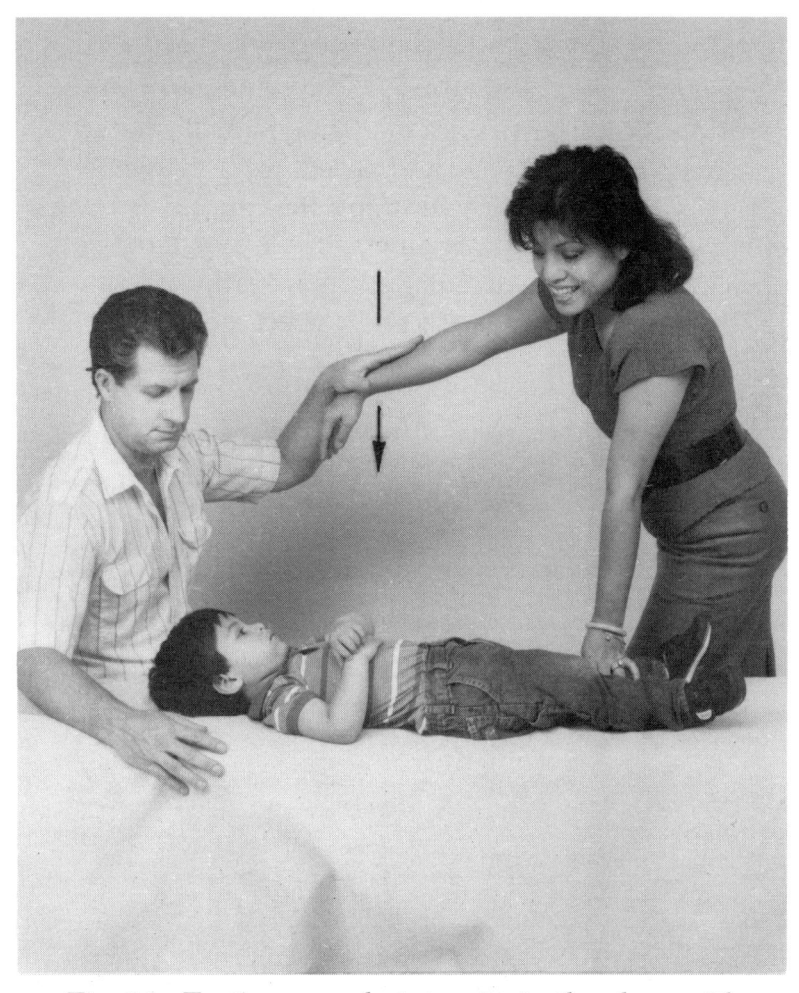

Fig. 16 Testing muscle integrity in the clear with surrogate.

CHAPTER VII: TESTING PROCEDURES

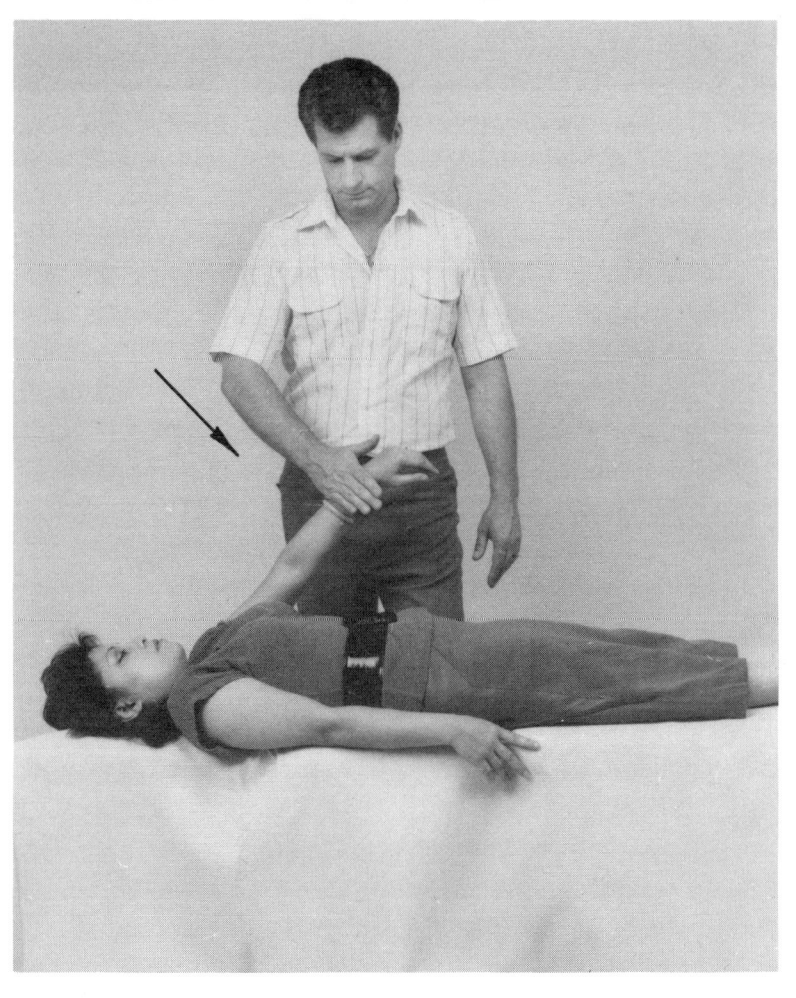

Fig. 17 Reduced testing angle for strong patients or surrogates.

# CHAPTER VIII: CHEST COLDS AND SORE THROATS

Chest colds and sore throats are often caused by the adenovirus—it may need a little extra persuasion to vacate, especially if it has already gained a foothold. The following procedure will be found to be effective. Usually you will be able to use "Your Cold Virus" through Step III and then implement the following additional procedures in between Step VI and Step VII. If "Your Cold Virus" does not access the bio-computer; use another witness.

For Example: On a blotter paper write "Your adenovirus", "Your Chest cold" or "Your sore throat."

The presence of cough, phlegm, difficult breathing, wheezing or sore throat will be your indicators. Apply Steps I through VI. If nothing surfaces in the clear remember to apply phase two and phase three testing procedures.

Remember: The witness was withdrawn after the liver correction (Step III) and not reintroduced until after the completion of Step VI. Here the witness will not be reintroduced until after throat/lung/bronchi corrections have been made. However; if you are obliged to change or use another witness (vibrational rate) in order to activate the bio-computer and implement cure procedures up through and including Step VI, remove the witness after Step III as usual-test and correct throat/lung/bronchi reflex points using Phase I, II & III procedures before applying Step VI . After Step VII reintroduce the witness and check your work.

First, have the patient lightly grasp his throat (parotid glands) as if he were about to choke himself. If the test muscle goes weak, you then touch the pituitary reflex point at the root of the nose between the eyes (Figure 3). If the test muscle becomes strong do the following maneuver. With the fingertips or heel of the right hand contact the glabella (Figure 3). Contact the occipital protuberance (Figures 2, 18, & 18.1) with the fingertips of the other. The occipital protuberance (inion) is the prominent bump on the back of the head. The head is cradled and as the patient breathes "in", the hands pull simultaneously toward the top of the head with even firm, gentle pressure. At the same time the patient curls his toes headward. The movement is as if you were trying to open a giant clam. This is done only on the in-breath and released on exhalation. Do three times. Retest. Repeat if necessary. Now touch the pituitary test point with the hand off the throat. If weak repeat the same maneuver without touching the throat. Retest the muscle.

If the muscle doesn't test strong upon touching the pituitary point with the patient holding his throat do not do this maneuver. Instead search out the spinal segments as the patient holds his throat and stimulate weakness as required. Generally the thymus is involved, if not the pituitary. In some cases both are involved. Check all three phases as well as other reflex points if required.

CLARIFICATION: If weakness while holding the throat does not respond in strength when the pituitary test point is contacted, then test other individual test/reflex points until you find one that does. Fix the organ per appropriate formula while the patient holds the sore throat. If a responsive test point cannot be found, then search out the spinal segments and stimulate the bladder meridian points with accu-digipressure where necessary.

Next touch the lung reflex points and test the muscle indicator (Figures 4 & 19). If weak stimulate the bladder meridian points adjacent to $T_{1,2}$ - $T_{8,9}$ - $L_{1,2}$. Then have the patient hold the lung reflex points and apply the same corrective procedure as you did for the liver/spleen/thymus. Also rub lung accupuncture points in a circular fashion (Figure 4). Next, sit the patient up and have him hold a knife edge palm (side of hand) over the bronchi (Figures 4 & 20). Test the muscle. If weak stimulate bladder meridian points $T_{9,11}$ - $L_1$. Retest. The muscle will be strong. Then have the patient hold the test point and fix all weaknesses in all phases . This procedure is also effective in asthma and other lung conditions. Where cough or chest symptoms are already manifest, this procedure can be repeated as needed until symptoms are resolved. Do only when indicated by weak test indicators. Check all phases and circuits.

You may have to test the bronchi first before the muscle tests weak. Check lung/bronchi or bronchi/lungs. The proper order is often required before problems are revealed or correction can take place.

Reintroduce the witness to the patient and test circuits A and B in the clear. If both test strong no additional corrections are needed. If either or both are weak recheck your work. You apparently missed something or your muscle indicator is inadequate. Remedy the problem as appropriate.

Occasionally excessive postnasal drip is the main contributor to bronchial irritation. It may be in concert with a violently running nose. If this is the case ask the patient to hold his nose as a point of contact while lying on his stomach. Use the hamstring muscle as a test indicator. If weakness is demonstrated fix all vertebral levels that give strength. Then break and reestablish nose contact & stimulate those vertebral levels that perpetuate weakness by contacting and correcting indicated accu-digipressure points. Next ask the patient to place his hands over the kidneys, palms up, as in Fig. 21. Using the hamstring as a test muscle indicator check for weakness., If weakness is demonstrated stimulate bladder meridian points next to vertebral levels $T_1$, $T_5$, $T_8$, and $T_{10}$. This is a phase I correction. Test for Phase II and III involvement and make corrections as necessary. Then ask the patient to turn the hands palms down over the kidneys as in Fig. 21.1. Test the muscle indicator. If weak, repeat the same corrective procedures as you did when the palms were up. Be sure to test for Phase II and III involvement. After kidneys are tested; hands are removed from the test area in Phase I correction and repositioned over the kidneys through Phase II and III corrections. These procedures deal with water functions in the body and their relationship to sodium/potassium balance. Significant distortions in these mechanisms often produce fluent nasal catarrh or stuffy states of congestion. Restoring a normal flow of energy to the meridians and related organs quickly allows the body to reregulate itself and reduce symptoms.

NOTE: Some individuals seem to "catch cold" or have repeated episodes nearly all the time. In these cases there is usually an underlying allergic factor that must be identified and handled if permanent benefit is to be obtained. Congenital miasm is also a consideration.

After performing these procedures gargling with

hydrogen peroxide (1 part to 4 parts water) or salt water is recommended. Do not swallow peroxide at this strength. It could be irritating. If a little trickles down the throat there is no cause for alarm. This serves to reduce infectious bacterial agents. Zinc lozenges are very helpful. See chapters on nutrition and homeopathic remedies for additional help.

By now the patient is feeling better. To reiterate; the best results are obtained at the first sign of cold symptoms. However, even if the cold has been evolving through the usual "ripening" process, application of the "Ten Minute Cure" will shorten the duration and lessen the severity of symptoms. Above all you must use Aconite and Nux Vomica to effectively conclude the "Ten Minute Cure". This is especially helpful for the cold that has been hanging on and refuses its proper place in oblivion. Anyone can catch a cold, now you have the technology to uncatch it.

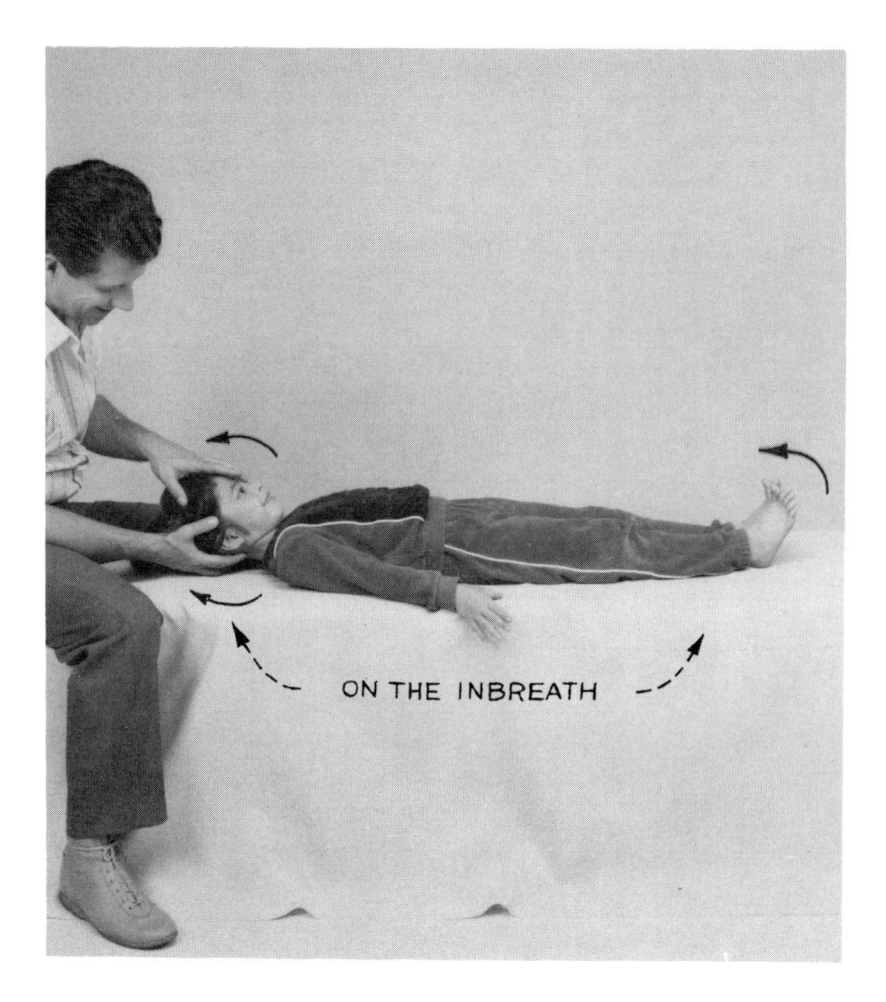

Fig. 18  Occipital/glabellar toe curl maneuver.

# CHAPTER VIII: CHEST COLDS AND SORE THROATS

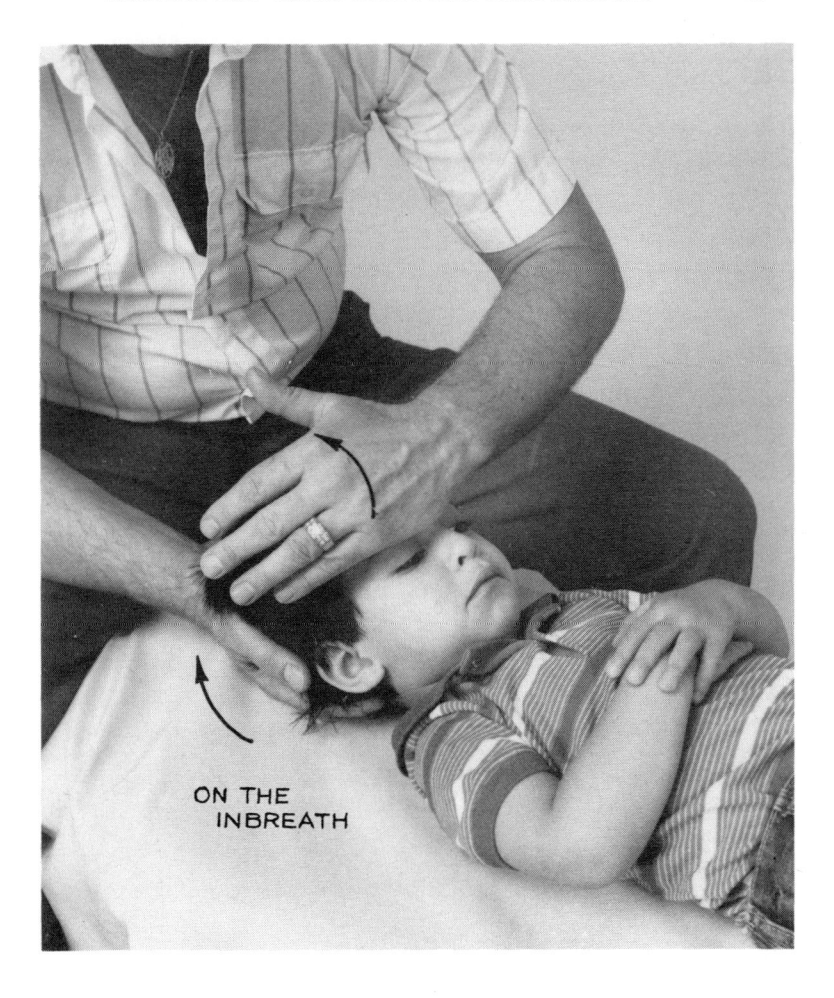

Fig. 18.1 Occipital/glabellar toe curl maneuver with alternate hand contact.

# CHAPTER VIII: CHEST COLDS AND SORE THROATS

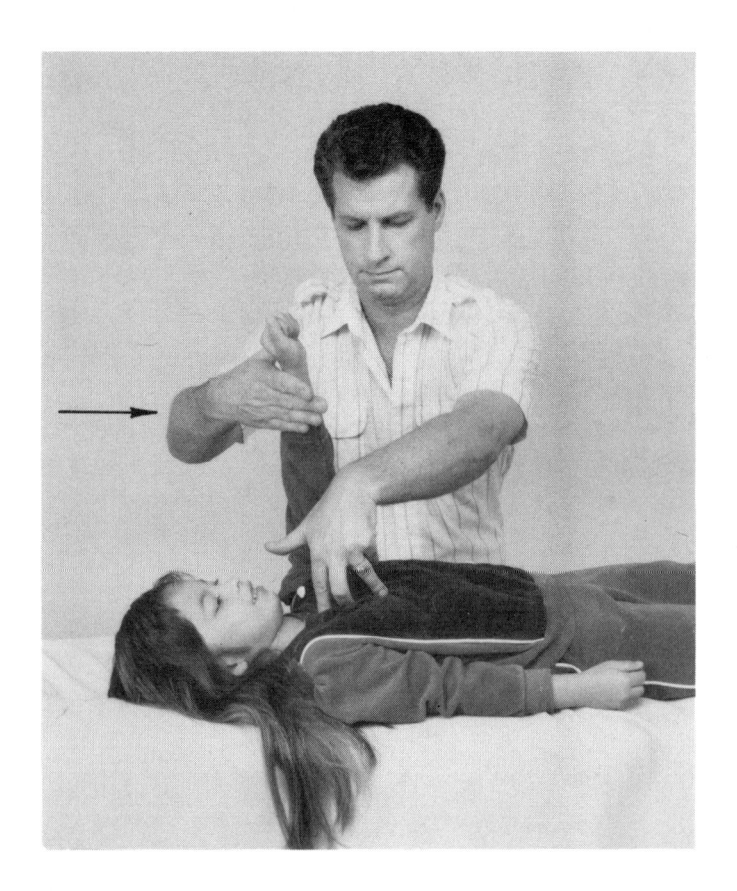

Fig. 19  Testing lung reflex points.

# CHAPTER VIII: CHEST COLDS AND SORE THROATS

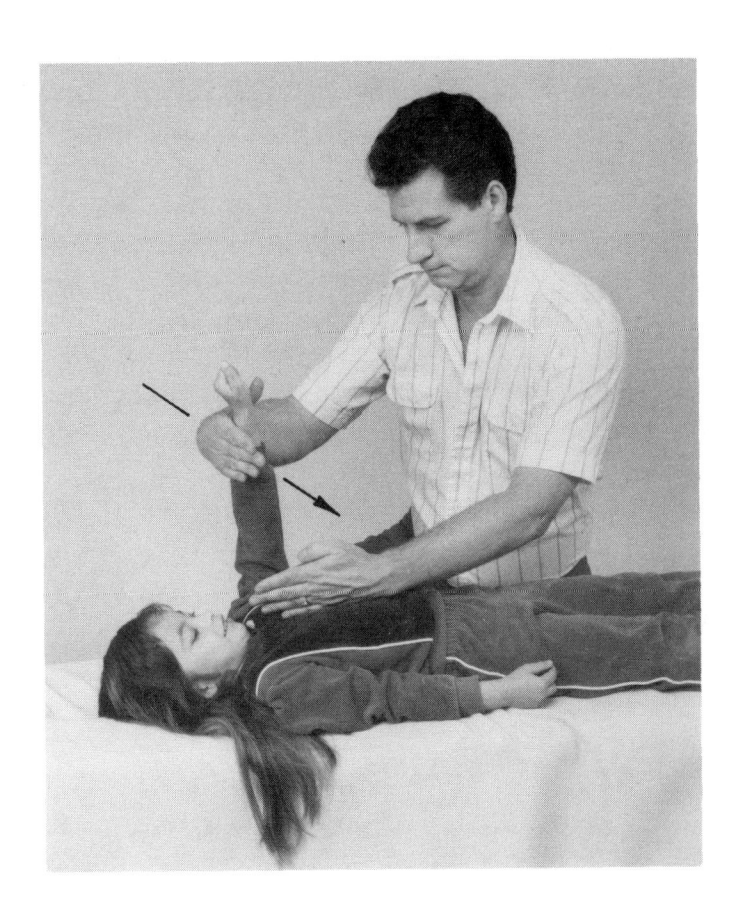

Fig. 20   Testing bronchial reflex area.

# CHAPTER VIII: CHEST COLDS AND SORE THROATS

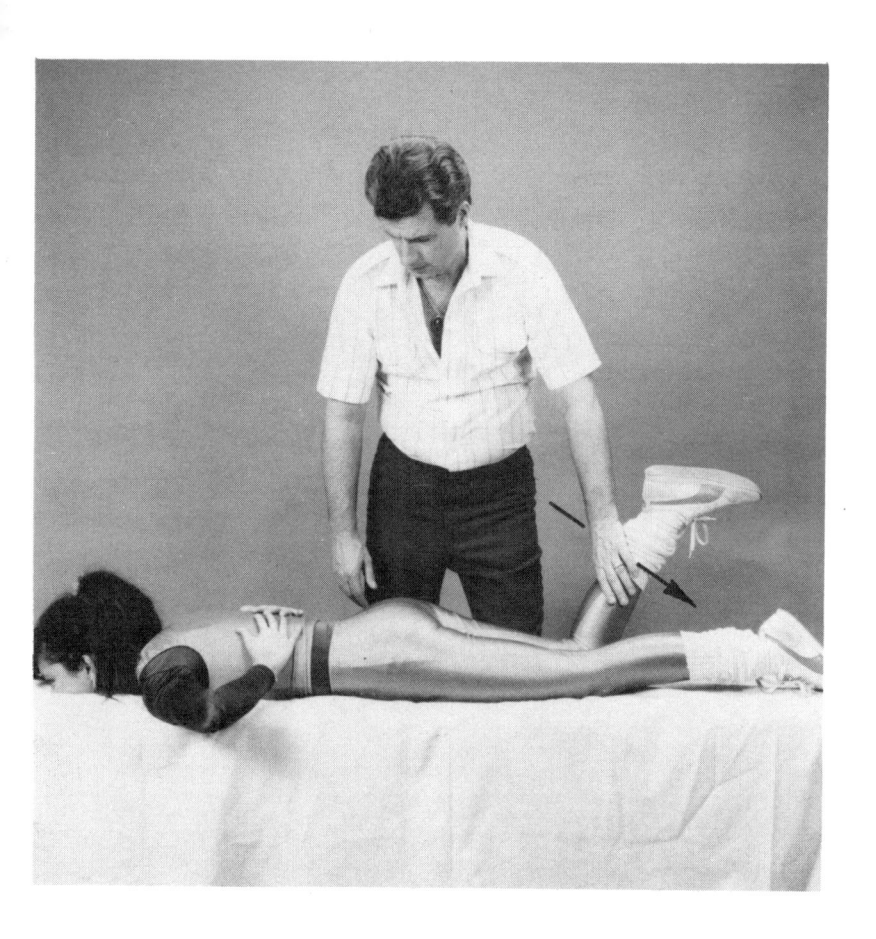

Fig. 21 Testing kidneys-palms up.

# CHAPTER VIII: CHEST COLDS AND SORE THROATS

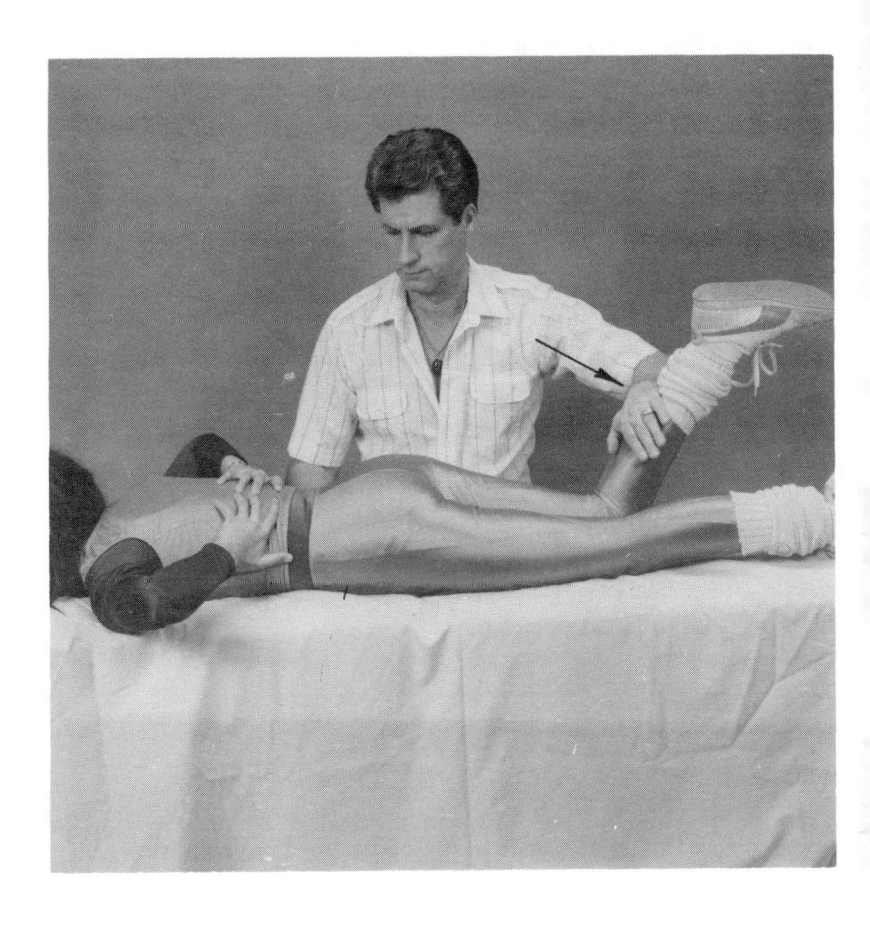

Fig. 21.1 Testing kidneys-palms down.

# CHAPTER IX: REFLEXOLOGY AND ZONE THERAPY

No discussion of treatment of the common cold would be complete without reference to reflexology and zone therapy. Almost every body function has terminal connections in the ears, hands, and feet. This is to facilitate transfer of Cosmic or Atmospheric electromagnetic energy in the case of the ears, or the Earth's electromagnetic energy with reference to the feet. Although the same reflexes are to be found in the hands and feet, the feet points are somewhat more accesssible. Your hands will be used to massage the feet and opposite hand in specific areas to ease viral cold symptoms. This discussion is limited to only those areas that relate to the treatment of cold symptoms. You may wish to consult other authors for additional information on these subjects.

A working explanation of this therapy is that the body is divided into ten zones (Figure 22). There are five on one side of the body and five on the other, both front and back. Applying pressure stroking to these zones stimulates any organ or body part located within these zones to bring itself back into normal balance. Every living thing must breathe or expand and contract to survive in a healthy state.

For instance, over a period of time the liver may become sluggish through viral invasion, poor dietary habits and improper emotional responses. The normal expansion/contraction process (circulation) becomes impaired. When this happens the reflex terminals in the hands and feet become sore and tender. This painful response is due to congestion or altered earth/body electromagnetic energy exchange. This body system stagnation process must be eliminated so that the body may once again regain it's balance of normal function. The pain and tenderness of the reflex points will then disappear.

How is this congestion overcome? It is overcome by precise application of scientific massage. This pressure massage is done with the tip of the thumb (Figure 23). There is a little knack to its mastery. It is not just a steady pressure but a slow steady creeping along of the thumb and retrograde motion or pull back. This can be likened to flipping up the cover and striking the flint strike wheel on a cigarette lighter. It is this movement that breaks the crystallized cellular granulations and restores proper circulation to congested capillaries. This is a popular version of how it works physiologically. Science may yet shed further light upon the true mechanics of this subject. It is reasonable to assume that this form or treatment has a beneficial effect on the accupuncture meridian points as well.

The question arises: Why does it hurt so much? Pain if viewed in proper perspective is really our friend. It alerts us that all is not well. In this case it becomes a test indicator. The places that hurt will be the very same ones that will initiate response to treatment. Generally speaking, the more an area hurts the more work it needs. As the pain response diminishes through treatment, body improvement accelerates.

The usual areas involved with colds are the head, eyes, ears, nose, throat, sinuses, lungs, bronchial tubes and lymph glands. Familiarize yourself with (Figures 24 thru 27). These are the areas to which you will apply scientific systematic pressure massage.

How much pressure should be used? The rule of thumb, no pun intended, is to use as much pressure as the patient can stand without bruising the tissue. It may seem that only a small amount of pressure may cause a lot of pain. Persevere—the results are well worth it!

There is an old Eastern proverb that states: "where the mind is; pain is—where the mind is not, there can be no pain." That is to say that the perception of pain is quite subjective and relative to the presence of mind. Therefore, when you experience pain while undergoing treatment it helps to concentrate on rhythmic breathing or take a mental vacation to your favorite holiday spot. Concentrate on anything but the pain. Pain thresholds vary greatly from person to person.

How long and how often should treatment be administered? Five or ten minutes after the "Ten Minute Cure" is applied should suffice. If clogged sinuses and eustachian tubes or sore throat persist, repeat for a couple of days until reflex spots are no longer "hot." If you find other sore spots in the foot while treating cold points go ahead and massage them too. It can only benefit the overall health condition. After treatment the feet will feel wonderfully warm and tingly. A good fifteen minute soak in epsom salts is also a delight. It helps to draw out the impurities you have broken-up and restore circulation.

## SPECIAL ZONE THERAPY TECHNIQUE

In rare cases even after the "Ten Minute Cure" has been applied and the foot and hand reflex points have been massaged, the nose and/or eyes will continue to run or paroxysms of sneezing may persist. What to do? Keep on hand a set of eight medium size rubber bands, or eight large clothes pins. When trouble persists within a zone, wrap tightly or clip the clothes pin on the ends of the fingers and toes of the appropriate zone(s) represented by each. In this case the thumb/large toe and index finger/2nd toe combination would be selected. They should be left on no longer than 20 minutes and care should be taken to be sure circulation is not cut off totally. Purple toes or fingertips are colorful but not desirable. If this occurs, remove bands and clothes pins at once until circulation is restored. Re-apply as necessary (Figure 28). This can be done with a piece of string or twine. Should the ears be clogged, aching, or discharging, shift therapy to the appropriate toes and fingers indicated in the diagrams (fingers/toes 4 & 5).

Treatment Sequence:

1. Do the bottom of both feet including kidney and adrenal points.

2. Do the back of both hands including Li4 located in web of both hands.

3. Do palms of both hands.

4. Do the top of both feet.

5. Massage zones on the outgoing breath.

## CHAPTER IX: REFLEXOLOGY AND ZONE THERAPY

6. Apply bands or clips to appropriate zones as needed.

7. Repeat any or all parts of the process daily as needed.

If extensive work is done on the feet and the overall condition of the body is in poor balance, a period of toxic cleansing is in order. After treatment, one may feel temporarily out of sorts and should immediately implement dietary suggestions covered in the chapter on nutrition. The final outcome will be beneficial. Do not expect zone therapy to resolve advanced pathological conditions. For these it is always best to consult a qualified physician. I do not agree with the axiom, "it is a fool who is his own doctor." However, it is wise to know when you are over your head and should defer to a professional.

Conditions like strep throat (high fever, sore throat, and swollen glands without nasal symptoms) or mycoplasmic infections (dry hacking irritating cough which does not relent) should receive medical attention. Upper respiratory infections may go into pneumonia and require antibiotic therapy. Strep infections are precursors of rheumatic and scarlet fever and should be handled without delay.

If symptoms do not rapidly abate or should they worsen over a 72-hour period, see your doctor immediately!

86   CHAPTER IX: REFLEXOLOGY AND ZONE THERAPY

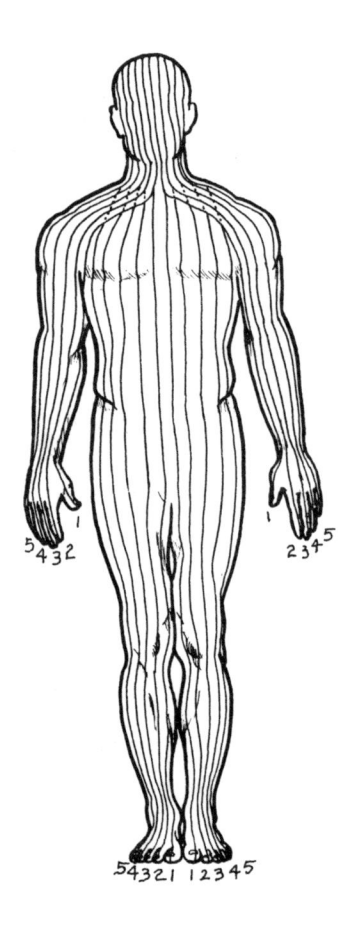

Fig. 22     Ten zone body diagram.

CHAPTER IX: REFLEXOLOGY AND ZONE THERAPY 87

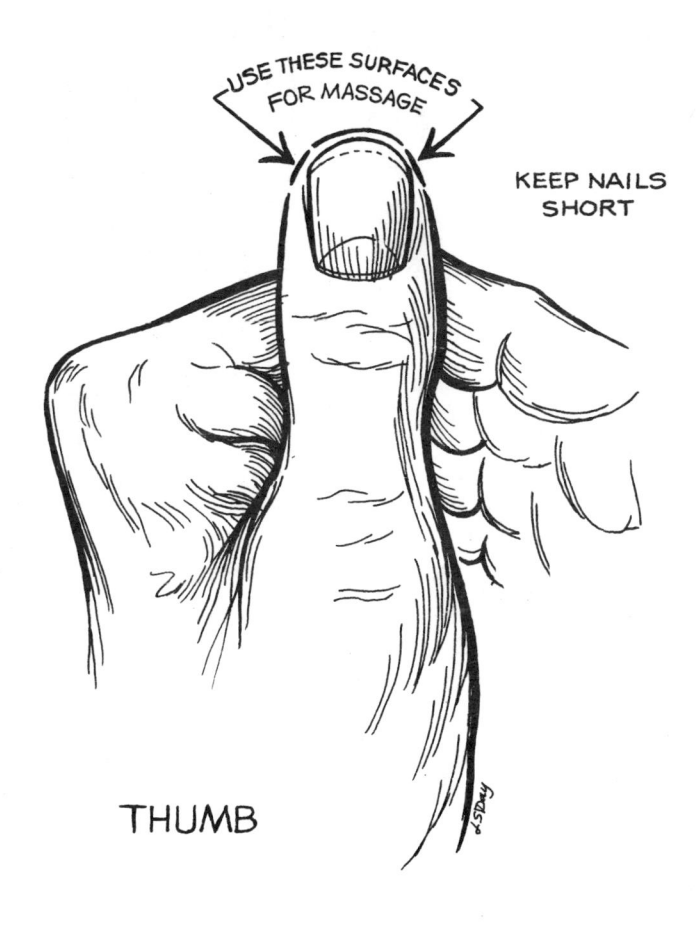

USE THESE SURFACES FOR MASSAGE

KEEP NAILS SHORT

THUMB

Fig. 23    Appropriate surface for thumb massage technique.

## CHAPTER IX: REFLEXOLOGY AND ZONE THERAPY

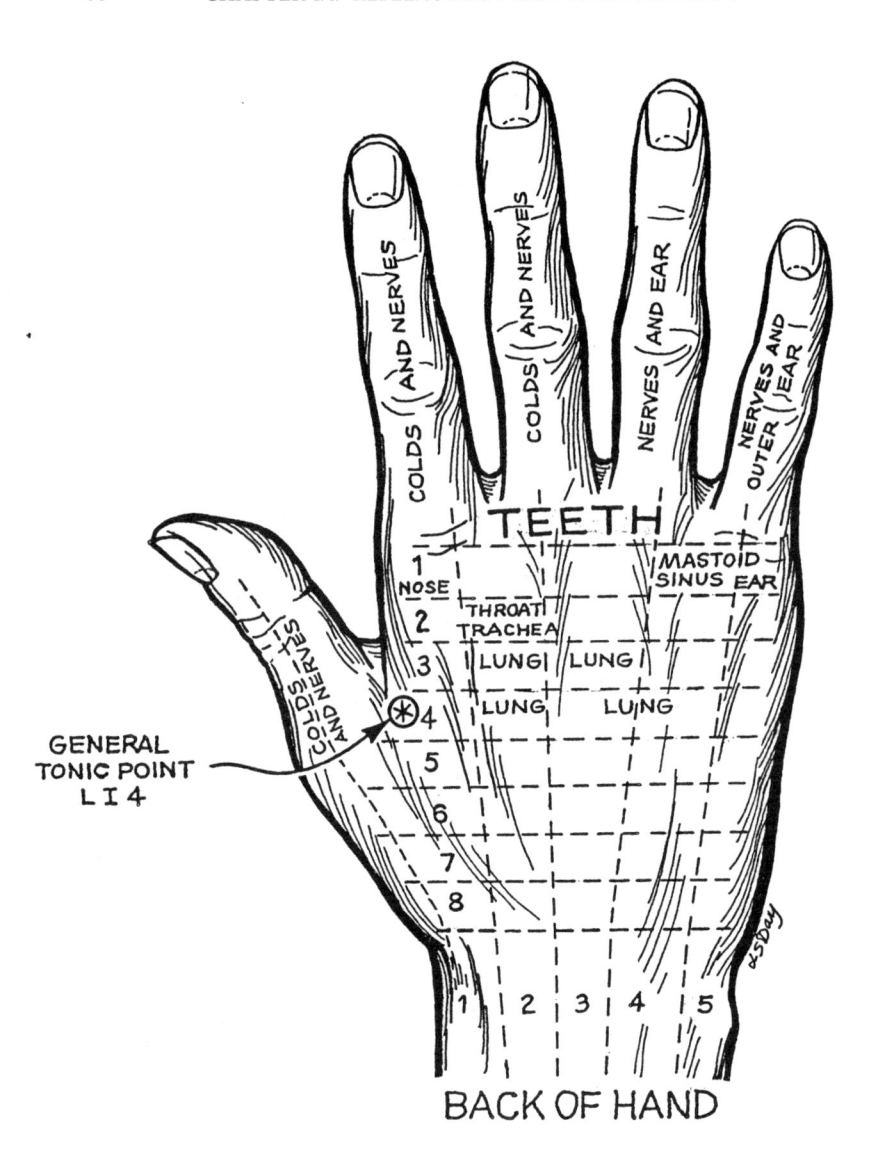

Fig. 24   Zones - back of the hand.

**CHAPTER IX: REFLEXOLOGY AND ZONE THERAPY** 89

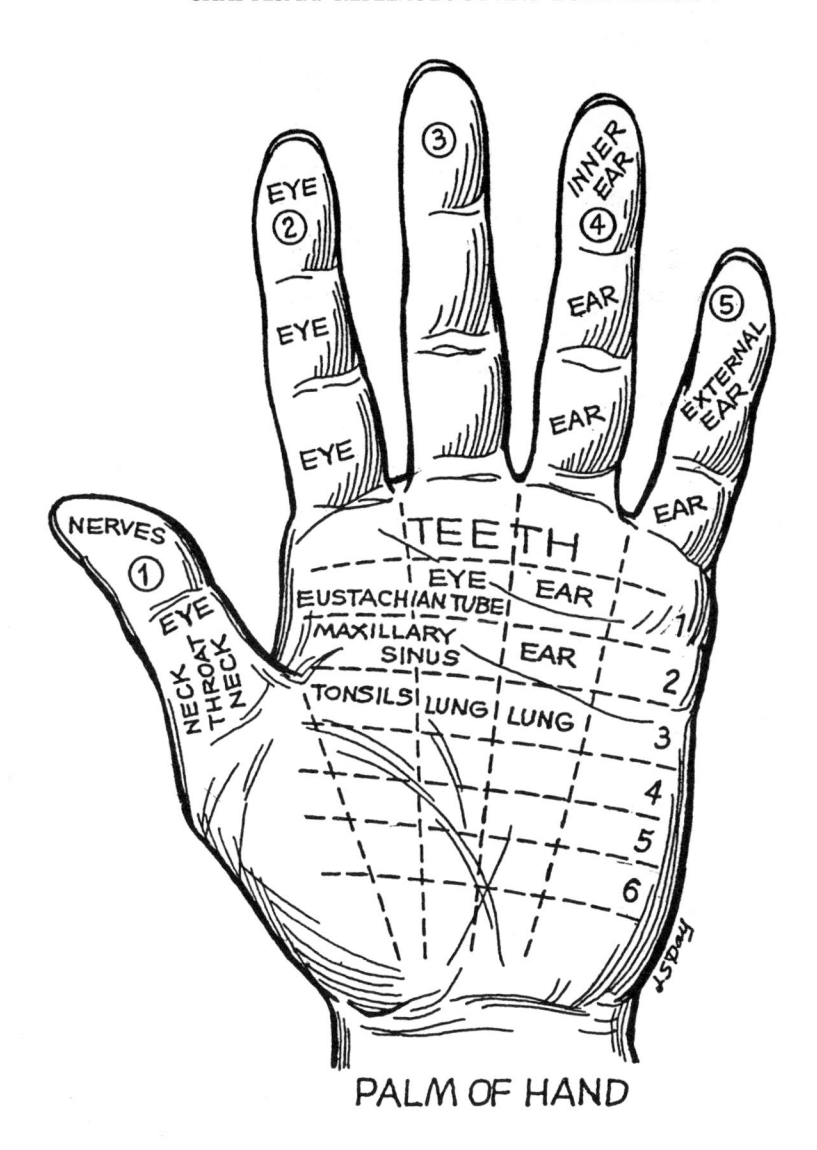

Fig. 25    Zones - palm of the hand.

# CHAPTER IX: REFLEXOLOGY AND ZONE THERAPY

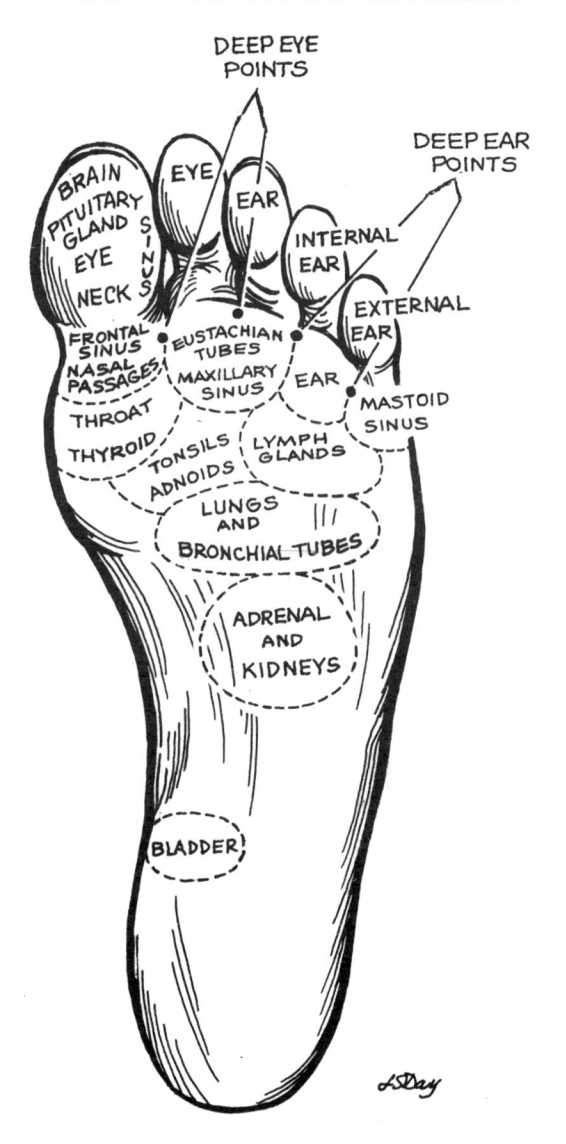

Fig. 26  Zones - bottom of feet.

# CHAPTER IX: REFLEXOLOGY AND ZONE THERAPY

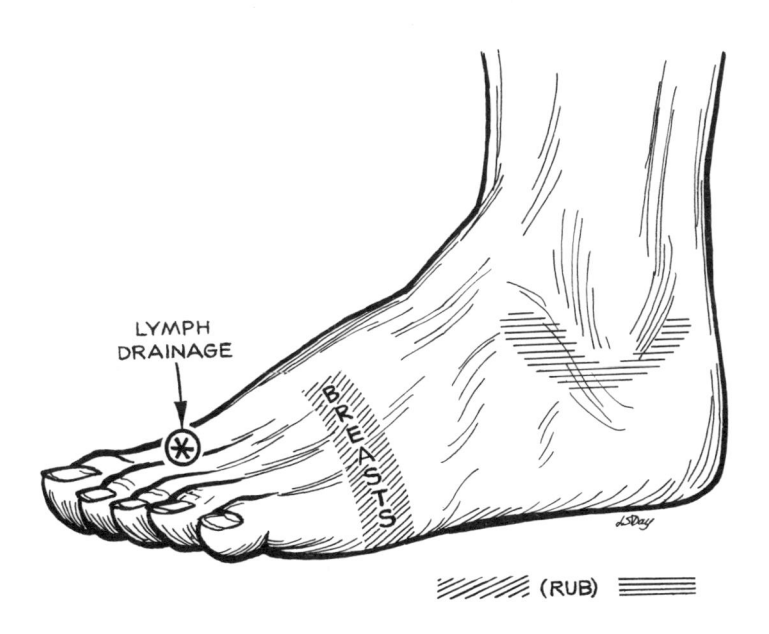

Fig. 27    Zones - top of feet and ankles.

92  CHAPTER IX: REFLEXOLOGY AND ZONE THERAPY

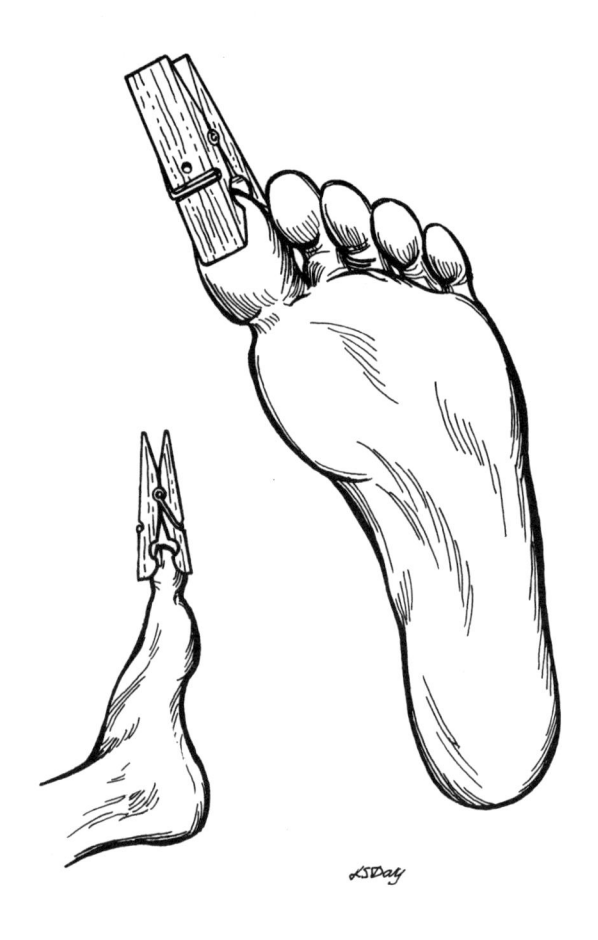

Fig. 28  Where and how to apply toe clips/rubberbands.

CHAPTER IX: REFLEXOLOGY AND ZONE THERAPY 93

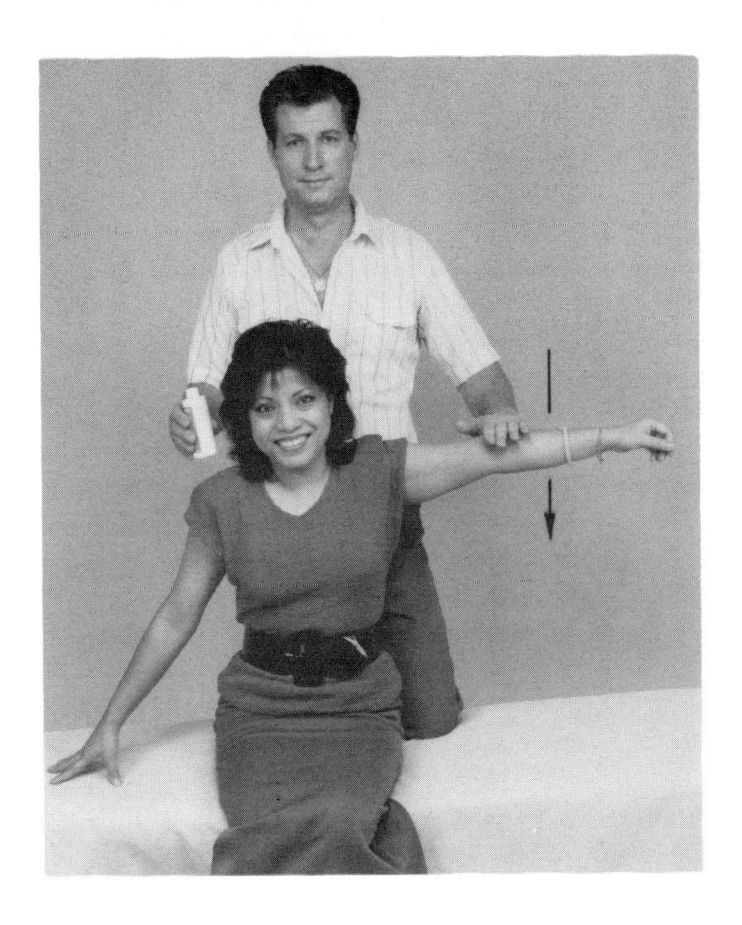

Fig. 29   Testing remedies using ear sensitivity.

# CHAPTER X: NUTRITIONAL SUGGESTIONS

During and after a cold certain food items should be avoided: alcohol, sugar, white flour products, greasy fried foods, milk, cheese and dairy products, red meats, and junk food. Coffee should be reduced to not more than a cup a day. Swiss water decaf is preferred if coffee must be used. This process washes out the carcinogenic chemicals used to decaffinate the coffee beans. It also tends to cause less allergy in the body. Cigarette smoking of course aggravates a cold.

If constipated the patient should be given sufficient buffered Vitamin C crystals in water to open the bowel. If allergic to corn or fructose use sago palm Vitamin C or Vitamin C from tapioca sources. Water soluble Vitamin A, dry Vitamin E, Panothenic Acid, the Bioflavenoid Quercetin and Selenium are also supportive to the immune system. Therapeutic doses of Thymus gland and Spleen strengthen the immune response. Sublingual elemental Zinc in lozenge form is antithetical to virus proliferation and should be sucked on slowly at the first sign of a cold; one every couple of hours throughout the first day should suffice. If nausea occurs, discontinue the Zinc. Do not take Zinc and Nux Vomica together. They have an adverse reaction to some people. Use one or the other, not both. Garlic and bee propolis have natural antibiotic qualities and are useful against viral sequellae. Garlic tends to antidote homeopathy or alter a remedy's action. Propolis should not be given to those who are allergic to bees or bee products. The same is true of bee pollen. Concentrated natural enteric coated proteolytic enzymes formulated in proper ratio taken four times per day on an empty stomach can reduce inflammatory processes and give the immune system an immediate boost.

The proper brands and dosages of vitamins and minerals are very important and vary with each individual patient. Most labels read relatively the same, but what's inside the bottle varies greatly in quality and effect. Again, consult the body bio-computer by placing a sample of the vitamin in the patient's left hand and testing an intact muscle in the clear. If the molecular vibration of the substance is acceptable to the body the muscle will remain strong. You may also test by bringing the substance in question close to the dominant ear of the patient. This is usually consistent with right or left handedness (Figure 29). The environs near the ear are extremely sensitive to input. Do not touch the ear directly. If the muscle tests weak do not use the product. It would be better to try another brand. It may be that that particular vitiam or substance is not indicated for that particular person. You may also test dosage in the same manner. Conversely, homeopathic remedies will test weak in the clear if, acceptable to the body. This will be discussed later in detail.

The foregoing suggestions coupled with plenty of suitable drinking water, a day's rest and relaxation in a peaceful atmosphere, will bring about a balance of energies. Do something that makes you laugh! This is all important because it lessens the possibility of relapse. Laughter is the medicine of the soul.

After the patient has recovered he should be encouraged to develop a regular program of aerobic exercise or yogic health system, such as, Hatha yoga or Tai Chi Chuan. Brisk walking is also quite acceptable. It takes 90 days to form constructive habits.

All hostile micro-organisms prefer lower oxygen levels than the body cells require to remain healthy. Boosting the oxygen level revitalizes normal cells while killing virus and other pathogens. There is no substitute for proper scientific breathing. Most of us have to be taught the correct method of abdominal breathing. People who reside in cities with poor air quality tend to breathe in a shallow manner automatically. While this does reduce the amount of pollution entering the body, it also reduces the amount of oxygen available for distribution.

# CHAPTER XI:
# TESTING VITAMINS, MINERALS AND OTHER CHEMICAL SUBSTANCES

Test vitamins in the following manner. Place one pearl of water soluble Vitamin A or any vitamin or mineral substance in the patient's left hand as he inhales. You test the anterior or medial deltoid muscle or hamstring and it remains strong. You put two tablets in the left hand and it suddenly goes weak. This indicates that two pearls would be too much, one would be the correct dose. It may be that five or six pearls would be the appropriate dose—too much or too little serves NO purpose. One should take nothing into the body; food, vitamins or drugs without first performing this simple compatibility test. Dose requirements may change from day to day and subsequent retesting is suggested. Herbal remedies would be tested in a similar fashion.

Pharmaceutical drugs or other chemical substances may be tested in the same way to determine if the substance presented has any adverse effect on the biological systems of the body. This is done in the following manner:

Introduce the substance in question to the body's biosphere by externally presenting it near the dominant ear or in the palm of the non dominant hand (see Chapter X). Test an intact muscle. If the muscle indicator is strong on a phase one challenge proceed to phase two challenge. If no muscle weakness is demonstrated in either phase, indications are that the substance being tested is relatively harmless to the body or in fact may be beneficial.

WARNING: USE COMMON SENSE! Do not ingest any known or unknown substance just because you do not get a weak muscle indicator. All assessment systems have limitations as do individuals applying a given system. Never expose anyone to risk needlessly. Some toxic substances will test strong externally and will not demonstrate weakness until taken internally. These are exceptions to the rule and beyond the scope of this book.

However, if weakness is demonstrated in phase one, two, or three challenges, you may rest assured that the substance has or will have a deleterious effect on the biosystem of the person being tested. Animals can be tested in this manner using a human surrogate tester. Positive test results (weakness) indicate that it would <u>not</u> be in the patient's best interest to take this substance into the body.

If the substance which tests weak is a prescription drug, the indication is that the drug may have side effects that could be troublesome. In this event the prescribing physician should be made aware of these possibilities. You may not always be received in an open-minded gracious manner when you confront the individual, but there is no reason why you shouldn't state your case. When a "cure" is worse than the affliction, a review of clinical procedures is certainly warranted.

In a crisis or life threatening situation, preservation of the organism takes precedence over any other consideration. Side effects must often be tolerated on a short term basis to accomplish this end.

An interesting experiment that you may wish to perform is to test a sample from your local municipal water supply and see how the body reacts to it. The results are often very suprising to those who are under the impression that tap water is generally fit for human consumption. Water supplies must be cleaned up or additionally filtered and oxygenated if optimum health is to be an achievable personal goal. Everyone should install a good quality water filter on lines used for drinking and cooking. See Chapter XVI for information.

Once you have tested each substance to be ingested, test all substances together. Often what may be acceptable to the body individually may not be collectively. You will be called upon to decide which substance(s) to omit.

By identifying and avoiding chemical incompatibilities when choosing potential healing agents, you will save the body from needless adverse reactions or side effects. Many a person has prematurely "met his maker" from inappropriate administration of well intended but lethal chemical combinations that were better left in the bottle in which they were packaged.

Another interesting experiment may be performed to determine the effects that heavy power lines have on the body's energy field. Muscle test any individual standing in the vicinity of a power line complex. The general response is extreme weakness. It is recommended that you locate your residence away from power line complexes or relay stations. These types of energies tend to weaken the immune system making it more vulnerable to infection by disrupting normal body polarity.

# CHAPTER XII: HELPFUL HOMEOPATHIC REMEDIES

The "Ten Minute Cure" is specifically effective in viral caused illness. However, in some patients the disease process can continue even after the virus has been put out of action. The following analogy may be helpful to understand the role of homeopathic remedies in this form of illness.

Assume that there is a match, and a long fuse which is attached to a stick of dynamite. In illness we usually find a primary causative agent, which in this instance is the virus. The process of illness is set up by this agent.

In this analogy, the match corresponds to the virus, the fuse to the development of the illness, and the stick of dynamite to the chronicity of the illness which has the potential within to culminate in death.

Dynamite will not explode if one immediately extinguishes the match which could light the fuse. Correspondingly, if one annihilates the causative virus factor as quickly as possible, the illness need not progress to the chronic state. However if one does not extinguish the match (destroy the virus) soon enough and if the fuse has been lit, attention must be focused on the fuse and not the match. Even though the "Ten Minute Cure" has dispatched the virus, the virus may have created a disease process which must be stopped, otherwise the illness becomes chronic. This is where homeopathic remedies become very effective agents in aborting the acute illness process. They are equally effective in chronic illnesses.

I will, later in this chapter, briefly describe the nature of these remedies and how to apply them. A word of explanation here is appropriate. First, these remedies are very powerful even though they may be highly diluted. Second, our knowledge of these remedies was obtained through clinical experimentation. In other words, practice preceded theory. Homeopathic remedies are vindicated by their results; even domestic and farm animals respond favorably to these remedies. This tends to rule out the "Placebo Theory."

Homeopathic potencies are identified by the letter "X" or "C" after the number of dilutions the remedy has undergone (i.e. Aconite 30X). This means Aconite has been diluted and processed thirty times and that it has a potency of 30X. Think of potencies as vibrational levels. It's rather like being in a 30 story apartment building where the sick patient is locked in on the 12th floor. Paramedics can't help him by going to the 13th floor. So it is with potencies. If the key to the lock is 12X, then 6X or 30X will be inappropriate.

This doesn't necessarily mean that a 6X or 30X might not be partially helpful. What it does mean is that the 12X would have a much greater effect and would perhaps cure when the other potencies may only ameliorate or lessen symptoms.

To simplify matters and give a point of entry to the

process of selecting the proper remedy(s), consult the following abbreviated Materia Medica. Choose the remedy(s) whose description or signature most closely resembles the patient's condition. Having done so, proceed with the muscle testing procedures previously outlined. To determine if one or more of the proposed remedies are acceptable to the body, test them individually and collectively for compatibility, potency and dosage intervals.

Remember the guiding principle "LIKE CURES LIKE." A healthy person given toxic doses of a remedy would eventually develop certain symptoms. A sick person with identical symptoms (never having taken the remedy) would tend to be cured by the very same remedy.

Remember: Homeopathic remedies will test weak in the clear if appropriate. This goes for potencies as well. The reason for this is that Homeopathy works mainly on the etheric body which is the invisible blueprint for the physical body. It is the discordent note that shatters the crystallized disease pattern that allows the body's energies to reintegrate. It may be likened unto the violinist who plays to the wine glass until it vibrates a such a rate it finally explodes. After this occurs harmonious therapies are applied to assist in total healing. Healing accomplished at the etheric level transfers gradually to it's physical counterpart.

## ABBREVIATED MATERIA MEDICA OF COLD REMEDIES

Aconite (Monkshood)   3/12/30X

> Take at onset of a cold... exposure to cold dry winds... eyes feel hot and dry but water-throat burns... chill... nose stopped up but still runs...

worse in warm room... restlessness and fearful at night.

### Allium Cepa (Red Onion)      6/12X

Sneezing, especially entering warm room... running eyes and nose... discharge "burns" nose and upperlip... hacking cough when inhaling cold air... better in open air or a cool room... catches cold in cold damp weather.

### Arsencium (Arsenic Trioxide)      12/30X

Restless, paces about... watery nasal discharge very acrid; burns nostrils, upper lip... better from heat, sore throat better from hot drinks... sneezes without relief... thristy but sips a little at a time... head colds tend to drop down into the chest... worse after midnight.

### Belladonna (Nightshade)      12/30X

Sudden onset... hot, dry flushed face... bright red sore throat... worse on the right... sudden fever... infrequent thirst... dry tickling cough worse at night... throbbing headache better by pressure.

### Byronia (WildHops)      6/12X

Miserable, wants to be left alone... great thirst for cold water... least movement aggravates... cold travels to chest... hard dry cough... chest pains with bursting headache... dry mouth but watery and/or stuffy nose... worse in warm room... better sitting up.

## Dulcamara (Bitter Sweet)  6/12X

Cold attacks when (weather changes suddenly, from hot to cold... nose, eyes run profusely... worse in warm room, open air... nose stuffs up in cold rain... worse in cold, damp weather... settles in the eyes... burning thirst for cold drinks... worse at night.

## Euphrasia (Eye Bright)  3/6X

Opposite of Allium Cepa... runny eyes and nose but makes the eyes sore... discharge worse at night, worse lying down... but cough worse by day, better lying down... eyes light sensitive and run all the time... feels better drinking coffee... worse indoors.

## Ferrum Phosphate (Phosphate of Iron)  3/6X

Beginning of cold when there is a slight fever... headache better from cold... feels as if sand under the eyelids... nosebleeds... coughs blood-night sweats... beginning stages of sore throat, inflammations.

## Gelsemium (Yellow Jasmine)  3/6X

Opposite of Dulcamara... weather changes from cold to warm/moist... dull headache; dizzy, drowsy... apathetic... limbs feel heavy... nervous chills... trembles... much sneezing, watery discharge irritates nasal passages... thirstless... better from urinating, open air, stimulants--wants to be left alone... a California remedy.

## Hepar Sulphuris (Calcium Sulphide) 3/6X

Colds develop in cold, dry weather... throat feels as if a splinter is stuck when swallowing... cough rattles... nasal discharge and expectoration is yellowish, smells like old cheese... extremely sensitive to drafts... very chilly... sour smelling perspiration... better in warm, damp weather.

## Kali Iodicum (Iodide of Potassium) 3/6X

Watery acrid coryza... facial neuralgia... pain in frontal sinuses- green bland discharge... tip of the nose red... swollen glands...brain feels enlarged... expectoration resembles green soap suds... cold settles in the chest... worse warm room; at night.

## Mercurius (Quicksilver) 6/12/30X

Very sensitive to cold... much sneezing... raw nostrils... yellow green nasal discharge irritates upper nose, upper lip... saliva fills mouth... hurts to swallow... breath and body odor foul, smells up room.

## Natrum Muriaticum (Common Salt) 6/12/30X

Violent sneezing attacks with irritating discharge... runny eyes... nose, either thin watery discharge or like egg white... stopped up nose, loss of smell and taste... headache... fever blisters... hates to be consoled... worse heat, noise, lying down.

## CHAPTER XII: HELPFUL HOMEOPATHIC REMEDIES

<u>Nux Vomica (Poison Nut)</u>　　　　<u>3/30X</u>

Give after Aconite... early stage of cold... nose runs in daytime, stops up at night...frontal headache... throat has rough, scraped feeling... nausea, vomiting... feels worse in morning... coughing brings on headache... hates cold air... do not take Nux with Zinc.

<u>Pulsatilla (Wind Flower)</u>　　　　<u>6/30X</u>

Use after cold has "ripened"... symptoms ever changing... patient cries, wants attention... chilly, thirstless... nose stuffs up at night, runs in daytime... cough dry at night, loose morning... lips peel... discharges of eyes and nose creamy yellow... better cool air, outside, cold food and drink.

<u>Quilla Saponaria (Chile Soap Bark)</u> <u>3/6X</u>

Most effective at beginning of cold... stops further development... throat hot and dry... difficult expectoration... sneezing.

<u>Sabadilla (Cevadilla Seed)</u>　　　　<u>12/30X</u>

Thinks it's seriously ill... dizzy... headache... spazmodic sneezing... lump in the throat... tongue feels burnt...chilly, thirstless... worse cold food, drinks, full moon... wants warm food and drink which relieve.

<u>Saponaria (Soap Root)</u>　　　　<u>6/12X</u>

Will often break up a cold... apathetic- depressed...

sleepy... head feels drunk...left sided facial neuralgia... eyes ache... runny nose... itching... sneezing worse at night... sore throat, worse left side.

## Tartus Emeticus
## (Tartrate of Antimony and Potash)  6/12/30X

Drowsy... weak... sweaty... down in the dumps... bandlike headache...child whines when touched... chin quivers... mucous rattles in chest but won't come up... low back pain... worse at night; cold damp weather; lying down. Cough worse after eating.

# RESEARCH NOTES

# CHAPTER XIII:
# HOW TO FIND AND TEST FOR THE APPROPRIATE REMEDY(S), POTENCY AND DOSAGE INTERVAL

Now having read the brief remedy profiles you will see that each has its own kind of personality or signature so to speak. The closer you match the patient's symptom picture to the remedy's sphere of action, the better the result. The cold victim need not have every symptom listed for the remedy to help.

Remedies of the most general use are: Aconite, Allium Cepa, Arsencium, Belladonna, Dulcamara, Euphrasia, Gelsemium, Natrum Muriaticum, Nux Vomica, Saponaria. When in doubt check these first.

The questions arise! How can I be sure I have a suitable remedy and the right potency? Can I mix remedies? How often does it need to be administered? In theory, matching a single appropriate remedy precisely with the patient's symptom picture would be all that is required.

In practice, you may have to combine remedies to get results. Remember that homeopathic remedies test <u>weak</u> in the clear if appropriate.

In this instance it is preferable to have a material specimen of the remedy on hand for testing purposes. This is due to the highly refined nature of the remedies. These may be obtained through homeopathic suppliers or from Sun Eagle Publishing.

METHOD I: Correct answers may be obtained from the bio-computer through muscle testing.

FOR EXAMPLE: Let's assume that you have selected Allium Cepa as the remedy of choice and you want to know if it is indeed the best remedy. Test your muscle indicator for integrity and place a sample of Allium Cepa 6X in the left hand of the patient and challenge the muscle. If it stays strong a 6X would not be appropriate. If strong, you either have the wrong remedy or the incorrect potency. Try other potencies. If still strong another remedy is needed. You may mentally, verbally, or in written form put the question to the bio-computer. "Is this the appropriate remedy (potency) for this patient at this time?' Responses: Strength-Yes; Weakness-No. It is only the homeopathic physical specimen that tests weak in the clear if appropriate. This is different from asking "yes" and "no" questions. Be precise; be consistent!

You may test combinations of remedies in like manner. Assuming Allium Cepa 6X gave you a positive result (weakness), and you wish to know if Gelsemium would enhance the overall healing effect, you would do the following. Leaving Allium Cepa on the body, introduce Gelsemium via the patient's left hand (right if left handed) and challenge the muscle indicator. If it stays weak it indicates Gelsemium would be compatible with Cepa. On the other hand, strength would alert you to remedy incompatibilities. You must test all varieties of combinations always discarding a remedy that negates weakness. Never use more remedies than necessary to do the job. If one will do it, stick to one well chosen remedy. Always verify your choice of potencies in like manner.

METHOD II: If you use a witness as will be described in the following paragraphs the muscle test will be strong for appropriate remedies and weak for inappropriate remedies. Use the system with which you are most comfortable. One can be used to cross check the other.

FOR EXAMPLE: A way to cross check is to put the cold witness/specimen on the body before the "Ten Minute Cure" is performed. Challenge the muscle indicator. The muscle of course will be weak if a cold is present. Now with the patient still holding the witness, introduce the remedy to the body in the usual manner. If the muscle indicator becomes strong, you will know the remedy will be helpful to the condition. You will no doubt remember that the action of contacting any reflex point (i.e. lung) becomes a localized witness against which appropriate remedies will test strong. You may also verify the correct potency and appropriate remedy combinations in this fashion. This should be done prior to administering the "Ten Minute Cure" because once done properly, the "Ten Minute Cure" will eradicate the cold virus, your indicator, and most likely the need for remedies. I have included remedies in this work because you will not always have the opportunity of getting an early shot at the cold virus. You may have to deal with progressively established symptoms which are viral residuals.

A word about remedy (potency) testing is in order. You may find that a muscle tests "kind of strong" but is a little "spongy" as it were. This usually indicates that a different potency is indicated for a better result or that a different remedy would serve more efficiently. Look for a more suitable remedy. If none is to be found, check to be sure the muscle has not become overly tired. With practice you will become proficient and with proficiency comes acute discernment. If unsure, test remedies in the clear using weakness as your positive indicator.

## HOW OFTEN TO GIVE A REMEDY?

The following method assumes the patient is holding the witness at the time of testing.

You may test the dosage interval by placing the appropriate remedy(s) in the patient's left hand (right if left handed) or in proximity to his dominant ear. Ask the bio-computer by testing the muscle. Questions may be oral, mental, or written. For example: "Should this remedy be given hourly?" (Weakness-No). "Every two hours?" (Weakness-No). "Every three hours?" (Strength-Yes). "Every four hours?" (Weakness-No). This last test confirms that every three hours would be most efficacious. In like fashion it may be determined how many days will be required to complete the cure. In some cases it may be appropriate to give the remedy every other day, every third day, once per week, etc... Do not get locked into fixed routines. The body doesn't necessarily function within static parameters. Again, be flexible and creative!

If not using the witness and testing in the clear, the indicator would be reversed. For instance, the appropriate remedy and potency would test weak in the clear. "Should this remedy be given hourly?" (Strength-No). "Every two hours?" (Strength-No). "Every three hours?" (Weakness-Yes). "Every four hours?" (Strength-No).. Again use both methods to cross check if uncertain. The subconscious will respond to almost any programming presented to it, but you must be consistent if you wish to avoid confusion within yourself.

Homeopathic remedies are generally given in doses of

6 tablets or granules under the tongue every 1/2 hour in acute cases (1/2 dose for children). Dose frequency is reduced as symptoms diminish. Absorption is extremely quick through the vast capillary system of the tongue and oral cavity. Do not take food or water for at least fifteen minutes before or after taking a remedy. Do not handle homeopathic remedies with the hands any more than necessary, especially the higher potencies. They are somewhat fragile and "fall apart" easily. Remedies should be stored in a cool dry place and kept out of sunlight, and away from electrical or magnetic influences.

You may find that a remedy may exhaust its useful action after several doses and will test weak or strong depending upon which system you use. Do not continue to give the remedy in the event this should happen. Probabilities are that the original dosage of the remedy was sufficient or if the patient still manifests symptoms, another remedy may be needed to complete the action.

If no other remedy is found to be suitable, you may let the matter rest. The body will finish the healing process. Never give a remedy without checking for body systems compatibility! The primary law of healing is: "FIRST DO NO HARM." With this in mind only good will issue from your efforts.

If this all seems totally confusing at this point, fear not! A professional quality videotape has been prepared to answer all your questions and to properly demonstrate all techniques presented in this volume. See Chapter XVI to order.

# CHAPTER XIV: CLEANSING THE NASAL AND SINUS PASSAGES

One normally uses these passages as air intake and expulsion ducts. The virus turns them into sewage lines. Sewage must be cleansed if order is to be restored. One of the best methods available is the "Nasal Saline Douche."

You will require a large mouth glass or coffee cup. Fill this with luke warm distilled water to which you will add 1/4 tsp. of sea salt. Mix thoroughly. Insert your nose into the opening of the vessel covering both nostrils simultaneously (Figure 30 & 30.1). Are we having fun yet?

Let the probiscus accustom itself to the water temperature before proceeding to the next step. Once accustomed to the water temperature curl the upper lip and proceed to draw the saline solution up both nostrils until it cascades down the back of the throat. Be sure at this point to close the back of the throat and expel the solution out the oral cavity. Do not swallow or choke on it. Draw the entire contents up in this manner. You will be amazed at how well your nose and sinuses feel afterward. Raw membranes exposed to excessive or iodized salt will burn considerably but not be harmed in anyway. Mix solution to tolerance.

An eye dropper may be used for the faint hearted. Tip the head back and insert the eye dropper. It does not work as well and takes a lot longer to accomplish the same end. Repeat morning and evening for best results. This method also works well for soothing sinus attacks due to smog, pollens or other infectious agents. Remember; "Practice makes perfect!"

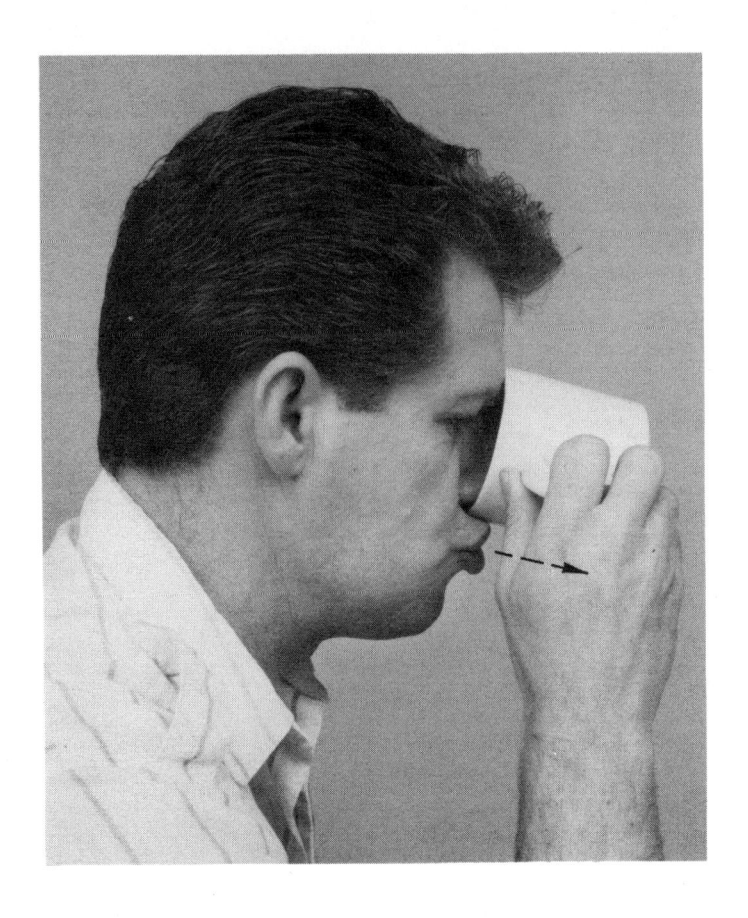

# CHAPTER XIV: CLEANSING THE NASAL AND SINUS PASSAGES

Fig. 30     Nasal Saline douche technique.

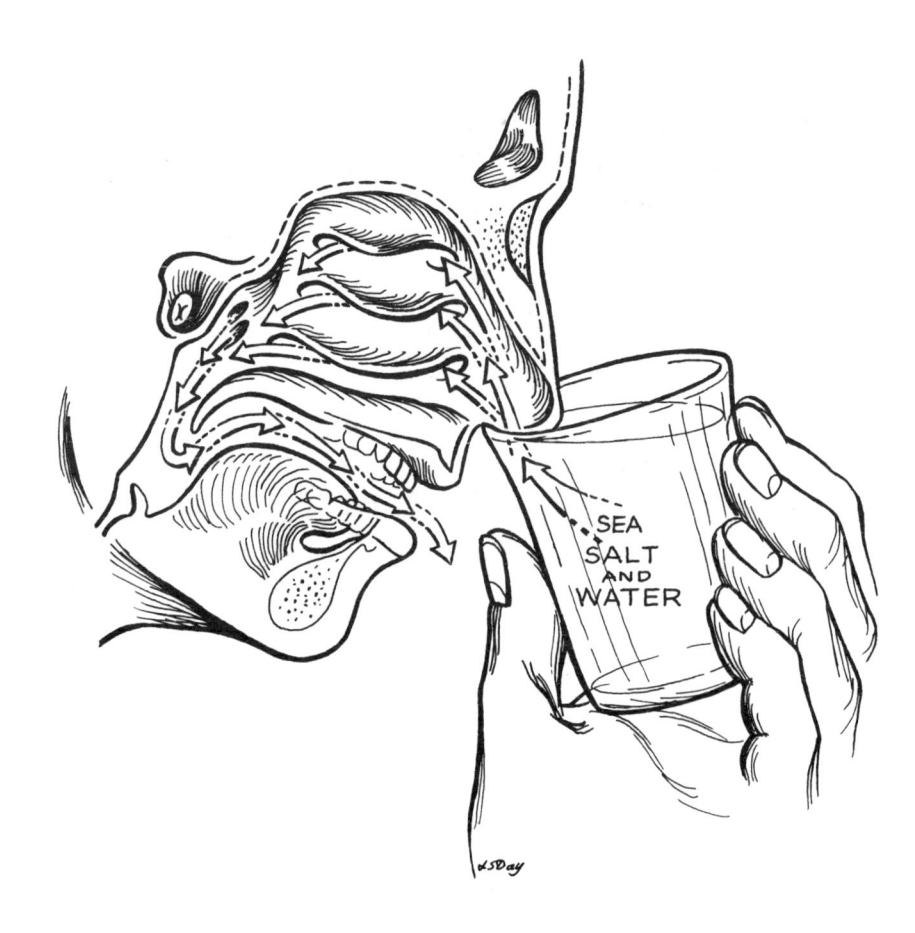

Fig. 30.1 Nasal Saline douche technique-internal aspects.

# EPILOGUE

# CHAPTER XV: EPILOGUE

I believe that all disease states are curable. It is only lack of knowledge and narrow mindedness that makes us prisoners chained needlessly to our miseries. Most of our modern technological and scientific achievements came to us from courageous men who were ridiculed, often punished and imprisoned by the "Orthodox Establishment." These men were no more than messengers of truths. Truth may be ignored, persecuted, and censored by the ignorant. Sooner or later truth always resurfaces at a more receptive time and appears to those who wear not the starched coats of contemporary dogma.

The proof of the value of any system lies within its results. To have results, it must be practiced. We are to use these techniques to reduce suffering, improve our health and the health of those around us. To do it justice, it must be practiced with a positive attitude looking forward to the intended goal—eradication of the common cold's onslaught. Do this with confidence! Do it step by step! Success will follow.

It is only in robust health that we are fully capable of achieving our fullest material and spiritual potentials. This is not only our God given right, but ought to be in my opinion, our primary reason for dwelling on planet Earth. It is not so much the quantity of life which is greatest of importance, but the quality of existence that matters.

We have all been given the priceless gift of free will. Should we not choose health when we have the means literally at our fingertips? To do otherwise would seem self-destructive. We must take full responsibility for our health and our lives on a daily basis if we are to arrive at any appreciable degree of self-realization in this lifetime. The choice ultimately rests with self.

James F. Dorobiala, D.C.
Granada Hills, CA 1988

**SELF HELP
SECTION**

# CHAPTER XVI: SELF HELP PRODUCT LIST

Dr. Dorobiala welcomes all constructive comments regarding the techniques presented in this book. Perhaps you will make additional discoveries in your application of them. All research contributions are heartily encouraged. Inquiries regarding educational seminars and public speaking engagements may be addressed to:

SUN EAGLE PUBLISHING
James F. Dorobiala, D.C.
P.O. Box 33545
Granada Hills, Ca 91344-8545

Available products for self-help:

**BOOKS**

A Ten Minute Cure For the Common Cold

## **Home Instructional Video Tapes:**

Colds (available in VHS and Beta)

Homeopathic Test Kits

Homeopathic Remedies

Nutritional Products

Water Filters

Write for details or call 1-800- 6 DR CURE
VISA/Master Card orders only.

# RESEARCH NOTES

# CHAPTER XVII: RECOMMENDED READING

1) <u>Time Magazine</u>, *Viruses* (pp. 66-78)
   Chicago, Ill. - Nov. 3, 1986

2) <u>Cure Most of The Ailments by the Power in Your Hands and Feet</u>
   D. N. Khushalani—Graphic Arts Press; Calcutta, India - 1980

3) <u>Materia Medica With Reperatory</u>
   W. Boerike-Boerike & Runyon; Philadelphia, PA - 1927

4) <u>Homeopathic Remedies at Home</u>
   Maesimund B. Panos, M.D. & Jane Heimlich; JP Thatcher, Inc.; Los Angeles, CA - 1980

5) <u>Spondylo Therapy</u>
   Dr. Albert Abrams—Philopolis Press; San Francisco, CA - 1918

6) <u>TBM Seminar Material</u>
   Victor Frank, D.C. & Hal Havlik, D.C. -
   Tujunga, CA - 1984

# APPENDIX I

# APPENDIX I:
# DIAGRAMS & PHOTOGRAPHS

| FIGURE | DESCRIPTION | PAGE |
|---|---|---|
| Fig. 1 | Bladder Meridian and Accu-digipressure Points. | 42 |
| Fig. 2 | Diagram of the spinal column, anterior deltoid/hamstring muscle/sacral base, coccyx correction points. | 43 |
| Fig. 3 | Cold, liver, thymus, spleen, pituitary, throat (parotid glands) test and reflex points. | 44 |
| Fig. 4 | Cold, sinus, lung, bronchial reflex points. | 45 |
| Fig. 5 | Testing body's natural antibiotic stimulation point. | 46 |

## APPENDIX I: DIAGRAMS & PHOTOGRAPHS

| FIGURE | DESCRIPTION | PAGE |
| --- | --- | --- |
| Fig. 6 | Testing anterior deltoid muscle. | 47 |
| Fig. 7 | Testing medial deltoid muscle. | 48 |
| Fig. 8 | Testing hamstring muscle. | 49 |
| Fig. 9 | Testing liver reflex area | 50 |
| Fig. 9.1 | Testing liver reflex area with surrogate. | 51 |
| Fig. 10 | Contacting bladder meridian points. | 52 |
| Fig. 11 | Thumb/pinky configuration. | 53 |
| Fig. 12 | Testing thymus reflex point. | 54 |
| Fig. 12.1 | Testing thymus reflex point with surrogate. | 55 |
| Fig. 13 | Testing spleen reflex point. | 56 |
| Fig. 13.1 | Testing spleen reflex point with surrogate. | 57 |
| Fig. 14 | Testing cold test and treatment point. | 58 |
| Fig. 14.1 | Testing cold test and treatment point with surrogate. | 59 |
| Fig. 15 | Testing sinus reflex points. | 60 |

| FIGURE | DESCRIPTION | PAGE |
|---|---|---|
| Fig. 15.1 | Testing sinus reflex points. | 61 |
| Fig. 16 | Testing muscle integrity in the clear with surrogate. | 66 |
| Fig. 17 | Reduced testing angle for strong patients or surrogates. | 67 |
| Fig. 18 | Occipital/glabellar toe curl maneuver. | 74 |
| Fig. 18.1 | Occipital/glabellar toe curl maneuver with alternate hand contact. | 75 |
| Fig. 19 | Testing lung reflex points. | 76 |
| Fig. 20 | Testing bronchial reflex area. | 77 |
| Fig. 21 | Testing kidneys-palms up. | 78 |
| Fig. 21.1 | Testing kidneys-palms down. | 79 |
| Fig. 22 | Ten zone body diagram. | 86 |
| Fig. 23 | Appropriate surface for thumb massage technique. | 87 |
| Fig. 24 | Zones - back of the hand. | 88 |
| Fig. 25 | Zones - palm of the hand. | 89 |
| Fig. 26 | Zones - bottom of feet. | 90 |
| Fig. 27 | Zones - top of feet and ankles. | 91 |

## APPENDIX I: DIAGRAMS & PHOTOGRAPHS

| FIGURE | DESCRIPTION | PAGE |
|---|---|---|
| Fig. 28 | Where and how to apply toe clips/rubberbands. | 92 |
| Fig. 29 | Testing remedies using ear sensitivity. | 93 |
| Fig. 30 | Nasal Saline douche technique. | 121 |
| Fig. 30.1 | Nasal Saline douche technique- internal aspects. | 122 |

# APPENDIX II

# APPENDIX II:
# PROCEDURAL FLOW CHART

I          Test an intact muscle
1. If weak, fix it.
2. If strong, prepare and introduce the witness.

II         Test the witness
1. Weakness indicates cold virus.
2. Confirmation: cold point tests strong.
3. Cross check: cold point weak without witness.
4. If witness fails withdraw witness and check throat reflex and correct if positive.
5. Reintroduce witness and proceed.

III       Test the liver reflex points with witness
1. If strong apply Phase I, II & III challenge and correction.
2. If weak check other reflex points. If strong fix appropriate points/organ as outlined.
3. Recheck liver.

| | |
|---|---|
| IV | Withdraw the witness from the patient |
| V | Test the Thymus reflex point<br>1. If weak, apply Phase I, II, & III challenge and correction.<br>2. If strong, apply Phase II & III challenge and correction. |
| VI | Test the Spleen reflex point<br>1. If weak, apply Phase I, II & III challenge correction.<br>2. If strong, apply Phase II & III challenge correction. |
| VII | Correct Cold, Sinus & Antibiotic point weaknesses by rotary digital pressure.<br>1. If still uncorrected apply Phase II & III challenge and correction. |
| VIII | Take Aconite 30X/Nux Vomica 30X<br>1. Administer one dose of each 5 minutes apart after the 10 minute cure.<br>2. Test for other remedies.<br>3. Testing may be done at the beginning before the 10 minute cure is administered.<br>4. If still negative, then remedies are not required. |
| IX | Test Throat/Parotids<br>1. If weak, apply Occipital/Glabellar Toe Curl Maneuver while patient holds the throat.<br>2. Retest the pituitary without holding the throat.<br>3. If weak, repeat the Occipital/Glabellar Maneuver without holding the throat. |

# APPENDIX II: PROCEDURAL FLOW CHART

X      Test Lung/Bronchi reflex points
1. If weak, apply Phase I, II & III challenge and correction.
2. If strong, apply Phase II & III challenge and correction.
3. Rub Lung meridian points in circular fashion.
4. Reintroduce the witness and check for strength (A & B circuits).
5. If weak check your work.
6. Do post nasal drip/runny nose technique if necessary.

XI      Test additional Homeopathic remedies for chest cold conditions if required.

XII      Administer effervescent bicarbonate of soda tablets or powder. Omit this step where contraindicated.

XIII      Apply appropriate zone therapy/reflexology techniques if required.

XIV      Perform Nasal Saline Douche as soon as able.

XV      Observe nutritional suggestions as outlined.

# INDEX

| Subject | Page |
|---|---|
| Accu-digipressure | 6, 23, 28, 36, 42 |
| Accupressure | 2 |
| Accupuncture | 17, 71, 82 |
| Acidic Conditions | 39 |
| Aconite | 23, 27, 28, 72, 104, 105, 113 |
| Adenovirus | 69 |
| Adrenal | 84 |
| Alcohol | 95 |
| Allergy | 2, 12, 15, 18, 27, 95 |
| Allium cepa | 106, 113, 114 |
| Animals | 100 |
| Anterior deltoid muscle | 28, 43, 47 |
| Antibiotics | 8, 12, 13, 20, 23 |
| Antibiotic point | 36, 46 |
| Antibodies | 16 |
| Antidote | 96 |
| Arsencium | 106, 113 |
| Aspirin | 23, 38 |
| Asthma | 71 |

# INDEX

| Subject | Page |
|---|---|
| Bacteria | 11, 16 |
| Bee propolis | 96 |
| Belladonna | 106, 113 |
| Bible | 63 |
| Bicarbonate of soda | 23 |
| Bladder meridian | 6, 9, 19, 20, 28, 34, 42, 52, 70 |
| Books | 129 |
| Brain biocomputer | 17, 18, 19, 31, 96 |
| Breath | 69, 70, 83, 97 |
| Bronchi | 20, 23, 45, 69, 70, 71, 77, 83 |
| Bronchitis | 1 |
| Bryonia | 106 |
| Candida albicans | 12, 13 |
| Capillary system | 117 |
| Carcinoma | 23 |
| Cervical segments | 19, 33 |
| Cheese | 95 |
| Chest colds | 38, 63 |
| Children | 38, 63 |
| Chiropractic | 1, 2, 12, 23 |
| Cigarettes | 95 |
| Circuits | 9, 32, 39 |
| Circuit A | 6, 7, 8, 9 |
| Circuit B | 6, 7, 8 |
| Circulation | 82 |
| Clothes pins | 84, 92 |
| Coccyx | 33, 43 |
| Co-enzyme Q | 39 |
| Coffee | 95, 119 |
| Cold | 1, 12, 20, 72, 95 |
| Cold test point | 23, 35, 44, 45, 58, 59 |
| Cold Virus toxins | 17, 30, 31 |
| Coronavirus | 31 |
| Cortisone | 24 |

# INDEX

| Subject | Page |
|---|---|
| Cosmic | 81 |
| Cure | 5, 27 |
| Disease | 11 |
| Detoxification | 2 |
| DNA/RNA | 16 |
| Dorsal-thoracic segment | 19, 28, 32, 72 |
| Drugs | 99, 100 |
| Dulcamara | 107, 113 |
| Ears | 83, 93, 96 |
| Electromagnetic | 17, 19, 81 |
| Electron miroscope | 16 |
| Enzymes | 96 |
| Epsom salts | 83 |
| Etheric body | 105 |
| Euphrasia | 107, 113 |
| Eyes | 83 |
| FDA | 39 |
| Feet | 81, 84, 90, 91 |
| Ferrum Phosphate | 107 |
| Fever | 17 |
| Fingers | 24, 84, 126 |
| Flu | 18, 28 |
| Fracture | 23 |
| Fructose | 95 |
| Fungus | 12 |
| Gall Bladder | 29 |
| Garlic | 96 |
| Gelsemium | 107, 113, 114 |
| Genetic | 17 |
| Germanium | 39 |
| Germ theory | 11 |
| Glabella | 70 |
| Hamstring muscle | 28, 33, 36, 43, 49 |
| Handicapped | 63 |

# INDEX

| Subject | Page |
|---|---|
| Hands | 81, 84, 88, 89, 99 |
| Hatha yoga | 97 |
| Head | 83 |
| Hepar sulphuris | 108 |
| Herbs | 7, 99 |
| Histamine reaction | 31 |
| Homeopathic | 1, 23, 27, 72, 96, 103, 105, 130 |
| Hydrogen peroxide | 39, 72 |
| Iliac crest | 20, 42 |
| Immune system | 11, 13, 15, 37, 39, 96, 101 |
| Inion | 70 |
| Joint lock | 6, 28, 65 |
| Kali bichromicum | 108 |
| Kali iodicum | 108 |
| Kidneys | 71, 72, 78, 79, 84 |
| Liver | 20, 23, 32, 44, 50, 51, 69 |
| Lumbar segments | 19, 20, 29, 33 |
| Lungs | 20, 23, 28, 45, 69, 70, 71, 76, 83 |
| Lymph | 83 |
| Massage | 82, 83, 87 |
| Materia medica | 105 |
| Medial deltoid muscle | 28, 48 |
| Meat | 95 |
| Mercurius | 108 |
| Milk | 95 |
| Minerals | 7, 99 |
| Muscle test | 6, 7, 23, 25, 28, 37, 64, 65, 71, 100, 105, 114, 116 |
| Mycoplasmic infection | 85 |
| Nasal saline douche | 119, 122, 123 |
| Natrum muriaticum | 108, 113 |
| Nausea | 96 |
| Nose | 83, 119 |
| Nutrition | 72, 130 |

# INDEX

| **Subject** | **Page** |
|---|---|
| Nux Vomica | 23, 27, 28, 72, 95, 109, 113 |
| Odic force | 17 |
| Occipital/Glabellar maneuver | 70, 74, 75 |
| Occipital protuberance | 43, 70 |
| Occiput | 43, 70 |
| Osteoporosis | 23 |
| Oxygen | 38, 97 |
| Panothenic acid | 95 |
| Parotid glands | 44 |
| Phase I correction | 7, 32, 36, 37, 72, 100 |
| Phase II correction | 8, 9, 34, 35, 36, 37, 72, 100 |
| Phase III correction | 8, 9, 34, 35, 36, 37, 72, 100 |
| Ph factor | 38 |
| Pituitary | 20, 44, 70 |
| Pneumonia | 1 |
| Polarity | 101 |
| Pollens | 119 |
| Post nasal drip | 71 |
| Potencies | 104, 113, 15 |
| Pranic force | 17 |
| Pulsatilla | 109 |
| Quercetin | 95 |
| Quilla Saponaria | 109 |
| Reduced testing angle | 67 |
| Reflexology | 81 |
| Reflex points | 7, 8, 9, 23, 24, 29, 32, 70, 82 |
| Remedies | 5, 27, 93, 113, 115, 116 |
| Respiration | 23, 24, 29, 32, 85 |
| Rhinovirus | 31 |
| Rubberbands | 92 |
| Sabadilla | 109 |
| Sacral base | 29, 43 |
| Sacrum | 42, 43 |
| Saline nasal douche | 119, 120, 122, 123 |

# INDEX

| Subject | Page |
|---|---|
| Saponaria | 109, 110, 113 |
| Scapulae | 20 |
| Sea salt | 119 |
| Segmental circuitry | 9 |
| Selenium | 95 |
| Sinus | 23, 35, 45, 60, 61, 83, 119 |
| Sinusitis | 1 |
| Smog | 119 |
| Sore throat | 38, 69 |
| Spine | 19, 20, 21, 43, 52 |
| Spinal nerves | 23 |
| Spinous process | 20, 52 |
| Spleen | 20, 23, 34, 44, 56, 70, 95 |
| Strep infections | 85 |
| Sublingual | 27 |
| Subconscious | 15, 18 |
| Sugar | 95 |
| Surrogate | 25, 51, 55, 57, 59, 63, 67 |
| Sympathetic nerve ganglion | 28 |
| Tai Chi Chuan | 97 |
| Tartus Emeticus | 110 |
| T-cells | 16 |
| Technique | 2, 25, 27 |
| Testing in the clear | 6, 37, 66 |
| Throat | 20, 32, 69, 83 |
| Thumb | 82, 87 |
| Thumb/pinky configuration | 7, 34, 53 |
| Thymus | 20, 23, 34, 44, 54, 55, 70, 95 |
| Tooth brush | 40 |
| Toxins | 1, 17, 30 |
| Toes | 84 |
| Truth | 125 |
| Universal Law of Harmonic Correspondences | 18 |

# INDEX

| Subject | Page |
|---|---|
| Vertebra | 6, 7, 8,9 , 43, 64, 70 |
| Video tapes | 25, 117, 130 |
| Virus | 1, 5, 16, 17, 18, 28, 30, 38, 40, 95, 97 |
| Vitamins | 7, 99 |
| Vitamins A, C & E | 95 |
| Walking | 97 |
| Water filters | 101, 130 |
| Witness | 6, 9, 18, 19, 30, 31,3 3, 38 |
| X-ray crystallography | 16 |
| Yoga | 97 |
| Zinc | 72, 95 |
| Zones | 84, 85, 86, 88, 89, 90, 91 |
| Zone therapy | 81, 84 |

## A PERSONAL MESSAGE FROM DR. JIM DOROBIALA

Dear Friend:

My goal is to publish timely, informative, health oriented, self-help books. You can assist me in this endeavor by answering the following questions, either by phone or by mail. If convenient with you, I would welcome the opportunity to visit with you in my office and hear your commentary in person.

- Did you enjoy reading this book?—Why?
- Would you enjoy reading another book of this nature?
- What idea or technique in the book impressed you the most?
- Are there areas of the book that you feel need clarification?
- Have you incorporated these techniques in your daily life?
- Have you discovered additional helpful information regarding cure of the common cold?
- Are there other health topics that you feel could serve as main themes for other books?
- Would you like to attend a "Hands-On" seminar instructed by your author?

If you have an idea for a health oriented book or videotape, I would enjoy discussing it with you. If you are already in process of writing or producing one, write or call me about possible publication at (818) 360-2224 or (818) 998-5087.

Sincerely,

Dr. James F. Dorobiala, D. C.

North Valley Chiropractic Clinic
17038 Chatsworth Street
Granada Hills, CA 91344

Sun Eagle Publishing
P.O. Box 33545
Granada Hills, CA 91344